Overcoming Commo

Coping with Stomach Ulcers
Dr Tom Smith

Coping with Strokes
Dr Tom Smith

Coping with Suicide
Maggie Helen

Coping with Teenagers
Sarah Lawson

Coping with Thrush
Caroline Clayton

Coping with Thyroid Problems
Dr Joan Gomez

Curing Arthritis – The Drug-Free Way
Margaret Hills

Curing Arthritis – More Ways to a Drug-Free Life
Margaret Hills

Curing Arthritis Diet Book
Margaret Hills

Curing Arthritis Exercise Book
Margaret Hills and Janet Horwood

Cystic Fibrosis – A Family Affair
Jane Chumbley

Depression at Work
Vicky Maud

Depressive Illness
Dr Tim Cantopher

Effortless Exercise
Dr Caroline Shreeve

Fertility
Julie Reid

The Fibromyalgia Healing Diet
Christine Craggs-Hinton

Garlic
Karen Evennett

Getting a Good Night's Sleep
Fiona Johnston

The Good Stress Guide
Mary Hartley

Heal the Hurt: How to Forgive and Move On
Dr Ann Macaskill

Heart Attacks – Prevent and Survive
Dr Tom Smith

Helping Children Cope with Attention Deficit Disorder
Dr Patricia Gilbert

Helping Children Cope with Bullying
Sarah Lawson

Rosemary Wells

Helping Children Cope with Divorce
Rosemary Wells

Helping Children Cope with Grief
Rosemary Wells

Helping Children Cope with Stammering
Jackie Turnbull and Trudy Stewart

Helping Children Get the Most from School
Sarah Lawson

How to Accept Yourself
Dr Windy Dryden

How to Be Your Own Best Friend
Dr Paul Hauck

How to Cope when the Going Gets Tough
Dr Windy Dryden and Jack Gordon

How to Cope with Anaemia
Dr Joan Gomez

How to Cope with Bulimia
Dr Joan Gomez

How to Cope with Difficult People
Alan Houel with Christian Godefroy

How to Cope with Stress
Dr Peter Tyrer

How to Enjoy Your Retirement
Vicky Maud

How to Improve Your Confidence
Dr Kenneth Hambly

How to Keep Your Cholesterol in Check
Dr Robert Povey

How to Lose Weight Without Dieting
Mark Barker

How to Love and Be Loved
Dr Paul Hauck

How to Make Yourself Miserable
Dr Windy Dryden

How to Pass Your Driving Test
Donald Ridland

How to Stand up for Yourself
Dr Paul Hauck

How to Stick to a Diet
Deborah Steinberg and Dr Windy Dryden

How to Stop Worrying
Dr Frank Tallis

The How to Study Book
Alan Brown

How to Succeed as a Single Parent
Carole Baldock

Overcoming Common Problems Series

Overcoming Common Problems

Is HRT Right for You?

Dr Anne MacGregor

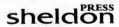

First published in Great Britain in 2003 by
Sheldon Press
1 Marylebone Road
London NW1 4DU

Revised editions 1998, 2003

© Dr Anne MacGregor 1993, 1998, 2003

British Library Cataloguing-in-Publication Data

A catalogue record for this book is available from the British Library

ISBN 0–85969–915–3

1 3 5 7 9 10 8 6 4 2

Typeset by Deltatype Limited, Birkenhead, Merseyside
Printed in Great Britain by Biddles Ltd
www.biddles.co.uk

Contents

Introduction

I was experiencing terrible depression and lethargy and had become weepy, getting upset and worked up about situations. But at the same time as worrying, I was telling myself there was no need to worry.

My periods were irregular, and I felt exhausted all the time – the frequent sweats meant that I never had a good night's sleep. I went to my doctor who said everything was OK except for hormone imbalance, and had I ever considered HRT? I had always maintained I would not interfere with my hormonal function but by then I was feeling so unlike myself that I was prepared to try anything.

Since starting HRT, I do feel better in myself, and no longer get uptight or weepy about things. I occasionally have night-time sweats, but they are not a problem. I also find that vaginal lubrication has improved.

However much we would all like to believe it, hormone replacement therapy (HRT) is not the secret of eternal youth, but it can ease the misery of hot flushes, sweats and sleepless nights that some women experience as they approach the menopause.

But HRT is much more than just a treatment for hot flushes – of greater importance is the evidence that if HRT is taken for several years, it can help to prevent heart attacks, strokes and osteoporosis (brittle bones), reducing the risk of death from these conditions by as much as 50 per cent. These life-threatening long-term effects of oestrogen loss are the most important reasons for considering HRT and are discussed at length in this book.

That is not to say short-term symptoms are insufficient reeason to take HRT; some women suffer considerable discomfort that may require medical treatment. In addition to having to cope with hot flushes, night sweats and feeling constantly tired, the change of life can be a difficult time, coinciding with stressful life events – retirement, children leaving home, death or illness of a parent. Most women adapt to these changes, but menopausal symptoms will not make it easy.

On the other hand, HRT is a drug and therefore has side-effects. Most of these, such as breast tenderness and bloating, are minimal and settle after the initial few months of treatment. If not, it is often worth trying a different type of HRT. The return to monthly 'periods' is more of a problem, but some regimes aim to avoid withdrawal bleeds altogether.

Knowing the pros and cons of treatment, and the different options available, are the key to successful therapy for any woman considering HRT. Unfortunately, few women realize the number of different types and regimes of HRT on offer. It is also unlikely that your GP or clinic doctor has sufficient time to go through all the options, side-effects and advantages or disadvantages of each treatment.

The problem is finding the relevant information that helps you make a choice. Only then can you decide that HRT is not for you, or vice versa. There are many misconceptions about HRT; in particular, its effects are often confused with those of the oral contraceptive pill. One of the major concerns about the pill has been that the doses of synthetic oestrogen, necessary for contraception, have been linked to a higher risk of thrombosis. In contrast, HRT uses natural oestrogens at doses lower than the peak levels reached during the normal menstrual cycle. Because of these important differences, studies show that HRT actually reduces the risk of thrombosis.

Furthermore, there are alternatives to HRT; non-hormonal drugs can be prescribed to treat hot flushes. Even simple modifications to your diet and lifestyle can make an enormous difference. Current medical knowledge suggests that watching your diet and taking regular exercise are important to your health, in their own right, regardless of whether or not you choose to take HRT.

Where do you find the information? Many of the books currently available on HRT have a tendency to be either strongly in favour of HRT, or against it. My aim in writing this book is to provide the reader with sufficient information to help her make up her own mind about HRT, and to understand the different options available. I hope that when you have read it, you will be able to make an informed choice which you can discuss further with your doctor.

I am not a gynaecologist so when I was first asked to write this book, I was uncertain about the idea. But as a doctor specializing in migraine and headaches, I see many women whose headaches become more frequent in the years leading up to the menopause.

HRT is often a topic for discussion, as irregular periods and menopausal symptoms are additional problems to the headaches. This meant that I had a working knowledge of HRT and its effects. But was this enough experience on which to base a book? I realized that my limited knowledge could be an advantage; as a woman, I will have to make may own decision as to whether or not I will take HRT in the future. Therefore I could base the book on my own learning experience.

What surprised me is the need to make lifestyle changes well before the menopause. In many respects, we have left it too late if we only start to think about the menopause at the time we are already experiencing the effects: although the risk of death from heart disease increases after the menopause, for too many people heart disease is merely a reflection of a lifetime of smoking, lack of exercise, obesity and a high fat diet – all of which can be changed.

Bone loss is the other major problem after the menopause. Many women are on a permanent diet in the battle to lose weight. Unfortunately, most dieters first cut out the essential dairy foods, considered to be high in fat, that help strengthen the bones, protecting them from fractures in later years.

So protection against heart disease and osteoporosis should start at an early age, long before the menopause. Even if you have already reached the menopause, it is not too late to make changes. If enough is done to keep the risk factors for heart disease and osteoporosis to a minimum, HRT may not be necessary. That aside, there will always be medical grounds for taking HRT, and the benefit to those women at high risk of fractures is indisputable.

Each chapter is complete in itself, so you do not have to read the book in any particular order, and you can skip chapters that you are not interested in. This is particularly the case for the early, more technical chapters which cover the normal menstrual cycle and the changes that take place in the body leading up to, and after, the menopause.

Sometimes the information may seem confusing; that is because, in many cases, there is no clear-cut answer. Research continually advances our knowledge of HRT. Some of the gaps have been filled in, but at the same time new holes open up; what is accepted medical knowledge today may well be out of date in a few years' time.

Included are quotes from letters I received from women describing their experiences of HRT. These tell their own story of some of the problems encountered and the benefits of treatment. My thanks to everyone who took the time to put pen to paper.

I hope this book will dispel any myths about HRT and the menopause. HRT is not a treatment for growing old. It does not affect the ageing process, and it does not restore fertility, but it can give enormous relief from the effects of oestrogen withdrawal following the menopause. Nevertheless, there are many other ways to minimize the effects of growing old, and there can be no substitute for a healthy and active lifestyle.

When the time comes to consider HRT, the choice is yours.

Introduction to the Second Edition

Since the first edition of this book was published in 1993, I have been running the menopause clinic at St Bartholomew's Hospital in London. I have enjoyed this immensely and am enormously grateful to my patients, and to the staff, for all that I have learned from this hands-on experience. It has been encouraging to note the upsurge in interest in the management of the menopause over recent years. This has led to the development of several new treatment options, which has made it much easier to tailor treatment to each woman's individual needs. We still have a long way to go to reach the goal of the ideal treatment – easy to use, 100 per cent effective, 100 per cent safe, no side-effects, and cheap – but at least doctors and the pharmaceutical industry are waking up to women's needs. HRT remains a highly effective means both of managing menopausal symptoms and of preventing against several conditions affected by long-term oestrogen deficiency. However, there are alternatives available. This new edition retains the original aim of providing information about the pros and cons of HRT, and the alternatives, in order to help you to make up your own mind about what is best for you.

Introduction to the Third Edition

Over the last few years HRT has rarely been out of the news. Results of scientific research have often created more questions than they have answered, particularly with respect to the different types of HRT that are available. While studies have confirmed the relative safety of short-term use of HRT for a few years, concerns have been raised about the safety of long-term use, particularly with respect to heart disease. This new edition discusses the results of this research in order to help you make your own decision about whether or not you should take HRT.

1

What is Hormone Replacement Therapy?

A woman seeking help for unbearable hot flushes and night sweats was told by her doctor that she had two choices for treating the menopause: either she took hormone replacement therapy and would eventually get cancer, or she did not take it, and her bones would dissolve. Fortunately the doctor was wrong on both counts. Moreover, the choice of treatment is not limited to one type of therapy: many different hormonal and non-hormonal treatments are available, depending on each woman's individual needs.

Why take HRT?

After the menopause, the ovaries stop producing oestrogen, and the resulting waning levels of this hormone seem to be responsible for the host of symptoms that some women experience. Different symptoms tend to occur at different stages of the menopause:

Early symptoms may start several years or a few months before the last menstrual period:

- change in menstrual cycle (initially less time between periods, then longer);
- hot flushes;
- night sweats;
- difficulty sleeping;
- headaches;
- palpitations;
- excessive tiredness;
- irritability;
- depression;
- lack of concentration;
- joint pains.

Intermediate symptoms are usually more of a problem a few years after the menopause:

1

- dry vagina;
- painful intercourse;
- loss of libido;
- urinary problems: leakage of urine, poor bladder control;
- hair loss;
- brittle nails;
- thinning skin.

Long-term effects may not become apparent until many years later:

- osteoporosis ('brittle bones'), increasing the possibility of fractures and collapse of the spine;
- increased risk of heart attacks and strokes.

What is hormone replacement therapy?

Hormone replacement therapy (HRT) simply aims to restore the missing oestrogen in order to reverse the effects of oestrogen deficiency. Low doses of 'natural' oestrogen are used, which is similar to the oestrogen produced by a woman's own ovaries. This is very different from the higher doses of synthetic oestrogens used in the contraceptive pill. Even so, HRT is rather an inaccurate term as replacing oestrogen after the menopause does not exactly restore the intricate balance of hormones to the pre-menopausal state.

What are hormones?

Hormones are chemical messengers that regulate the body functions. They are produced by a gland, secreted into the bloodstream and then circulate round the body. Certain tissues or organs in distant parts of the body from the gland are able to respond to these messages.

Imagine the way that a radio transmitter works; hormones operate in a similar fashion. A gland emits a signal that is sent to every cell in the body; for any of these cells to respond, their radio receivers must be turned on, and tuned to the proper frequency. There are many distinct transmitters sending out signals that are picked up by different radio receivers, each tuned to specific frequencies.

The ovaries act as transmitters. During the menstrual cycle they produce varying amounts of the hormones oestrogen and progesterone that are carried round the body in the bloodstream. The uterus is one of the specific radio receivers for these hormones, tuned in to the right frequency to decode the different signals. Other receivers are in the brain: the hypothalamus (the master organ of the brain) and the pituitary gland. Many other tissues in the body also respond to oestrogen, including skin, hair and bone.

As well as being a transmitter, the ovary is also a receiver, picking up signals transmitted from the pituitary gland. In turn, the pituitary gland itself receives messages from the hypothalamus, closing the loop between the three glands.

Short-term relief

The menopause is a natural life event that every woman experiences as she grows older, usually around the age of 50. It is not a disease, and does not automatically require treatment; not all women have problems. The menopause may just be the uneventful finale to regular monthly periods, with little discomfort. It can even be a time of enormous relief, when the blight from monthly pre-menstrual symptoms and bleeding is over.

However, some women have quite distressing menopausal symptoms. Oestrogen replacement can relieve the misery of hot flushes, night sweats, bladder problems and vaginal dryness which result from falling levels of oestrogen. Although estimates suggest that as many as 75 to 85 per cent of women experience menopausal symptoms, only 10 to 18 per cent have consulted a doctor. This low figure has led some doctors to argue that the negative aspects of the menopause are greatly exaggerated. Many of these symptoms resolve with HRT. An exception is that an irregular menstrual pattern does not always improve, as underlying natural cycles may persist and compete with the HRT, which is attempting to regulate the cycle.

Long-term protection

For many years, HRT has been prescribed mainly for the treatment of menopausal symptoms, but more and more doctors are recommending its use as a preventative therapy. They argue that oestrogen saves lives, and that there are good reasons to support the belief that every woman should be offered HRT when she reaches the menopause. Certainly, research suggests that low levels of oestrogen

3

in the body after the menopause can increase the likelihood of heart disease, strokes and fractures.

By the time a woman reaches her seventies, she has a 50 per cent chance of fracturing a bone because of osteoporosis. These fractures particularly affect the wrist, hip and spine. HRT prevents osteoporosis developing and so reduces the risk.

The extent of the problem

If HRT is so effective, why don't more women take it? Post-menopausal women now make up some 15 per cent of the population, a figure which will rise to 20 per cent over the next few years. With better health and nutrition, women are living longer. Over the next thirty years, the number of women over the age of 85 will increase by a staggering 50 per cent. Many doctors feel that HRT could make a significant impact on the well-being of these women by reducing the odds of their suffering from fractures.

Even with the weight of evidence in its favour, a recent general practice survey by the Medical Research Council estimated that overall only 9 per cent of post-menopausal women in the UK take HRT, compared to 80 per cent in the USA. There are several possible reasons for this difference: lack of information on the part of both doctors and their patients, fear of serious side-effects such as breast cancer and blood clots, and possibly also the more conservative attitude to new treatments that exists in the UK.

The menopausal syndrome: a Western disease?

Diametrically opposing cultural attitudes surround the menopause. Many women living in Third World countries welcome the higher social status that follows the menopause. They are the elders of the family group with their own defined set of responsibilities; they have fulfilled their social duty to bear and raise children and are freed from the taboos of menstruation. Not surprisingly, these women welcome the menopause as a natural transition to a role in which they command greater respect.

Anthropologist Yewoubdar Beyene studied women living in Mayan villages and found that they looked forward to the menopause, as it freed them from a continual state of bearing children. She also studied the Greek peasant women living in Evia and similarly found that they had few negative feelings about the menopause.

4

In contrast, Western culture depicts the menopause as a time of loss. The media are particularly to blame, as they place a great deal of emphasis on a woman's youth and sexuality. The natural process of ageing is devalued; picture the stereotyped asexual, depressed, menopausal housewife frequently depicted in the popular press.

Unfortunately, the publicity that the press give to HRT has encouraged misinformation. Many doctors are confronted by women who think that HRT will make them look glamorous and sexy and stop them growing old; not surprisingly, about one third of women who begin HRT stop treatment because it does not fulfil these unrealistic expectations.

Side-effects are another favourite of the popular press. In the early years of HRT development, a small percentage of women developed cancer of the uterus (the womb) when they took oestrogen therapy. This fact was widely publicized as headline news. Fortunately doctors found that a second hormone, progestogen, prevented the development of this cancer. For this reason, doctors now recommend that unless a woman has had a hysterectomy, she should take progestogen in addition to the oestrogen. But these reassuring findings did not command the same media interest.

The need for information

Women approaching the menopause need information; most do not know a great deal about what is happening to them, even less about the diversity of treatments, both hormonal and non-hormonal, drug and non-drug, currently available.

The pharmaceutical company Schering sponsored a survey about the menopause, carried out by *Woman's Realm* magazine. Of the 1,200 replies analysed, 78 per cent of women wanted more facts about HRT. A disturbing figure was that 83 per cent obtained most of their knowledge from magazines; only 16 per cent said that their main source of information was a doctor.

Whatever the true picture, there is no doubt that HRT is of great benefit to some women, especially when it is recommended on medical grounds. This is particularly the case for those who have had an early menopause or surgical removal of the ovaries; these women are at greater risk of heart disease, strokes and osteoporosis than women who have their menopause after the age of 50.

Unfortunately, lack of information and, worse still, misinformation affect any decision made about whether or not to start HRT. This means that some women who would clearly benefit from HRT miss out, and others take it for the wrong reasons. Added to this is the enormous inconsistency in the advice that doctors give to menopausal women.

Many women are put off taking HRT, or stop using it after only a short while: of the women who had tried HRT in the *Woman's Realm* survey, 28 per cent gave it up within a year, and over one third within two years. The reasons they gave for stopping treatment were side-effects or fear of side-effects, their doctor's advice, or the return of bleeding.

Unnatural relief?

There is a school of thought that hormone replacement therapy is tampering with nature. Many doctors disagree with this, arguing that the menopause is a deficiency disease, and that the post-menopausal reduction in oestrogen is itself unnatural.

But it could also be argued that the menopausal syndrome is a product of the cumulative effects of improved medical and social care resulting in increasing numbers of women outliving their natural reproductive capacity. In 1850 a woman would live for an average of only 38 years, so most never lived long enough to reach the menopause. By the turn of the last century, life expectancy had increased to the age of 50. It is now about 83 years in Western women.

Treating hormonal deficiencies is common practice: doctors prescribe insulin to diabetics, and thyroxine for certain thyroid problems. Why is the treatment of post-menopausal oestrogen deficiency not viewed in a similar fashion?

Advantages versus disadvantages

The advantages of hormone replacement therapy must be weighed against the disadvantages; this balance is constantly changing.

Information about the HRT used today has been accumulating since the 1940s. Obviously, less data have been collected on more recently introduced treatments. This means that there is still a great deal that doctors do not know, about either the benefits or the long-term risks of HRT.

6

Advances in therapy have resulted in a vast number of different treatments currently recommended. These differ in the types of hormones used, and in the route they are given – tablets, patches or implants. There are also several different suggested regimes for taking HRT. The growing interest in HRT has increased the amount of research. The results of recent studies show that many more women would potentially benefit from oestrogen therapy than was previously thought. It has also helped us to identify those women who should avoid HRT.

The decision to treat

Although long-term studies show the enormous overall benefits for large numbers of women, they do not assess individual needs. There is not much point in a woman taking HRT if she has few menopausal symptoms and does not run a high risk of fractures. So how do you decide whether HRT is going to benefit *you*?

Imagine you have heard about how HRT protects against fractures, but have also read reports about the possible risk of breast cancer from long-term therapy. If you run a low risk of osteoporosis but several of your relatives have had breast cancer, you might feel that your personal risk of breast cancer outweighs the protective effects of HRT. On the other hand, if your mother is severely disabled from a fractured hip or collapsed spine, the protective effect of HRT against osteoporosis might, on balance, outweigh the risk of breast cancer.

With this information, you can tailor the treatment to suit you: the decision to take HRT rests on your individual needs, balanced against your health, lifestyle and family history.

As one woman's own story tells:

> *My GP is concerned about a possible increased cancer risk from HRT, since I had breast cancer – treated by mastectomy – 12 years ago. He prescribes HRT for me, with some reluctance, but is prepared to allow me the choice between a possible increased risk and a life which is impossible to manage because of the unbearable symptoms when I stop the therapy.*

Her decision was in favour of HRT; yours may not be. Either way, you need the facts before you can make an informed choice. For many women, the menopause is not a pleasant prospect. Few people want to confront the unavoidable evidence of growing old. Nevertheless, the symptoms women experience around the menopause are the result of more than just hormonal fluctuations; the menopause often coincides with a time of major life stresses – job responsibilities, elderly or ailing parents, and children leaving home. HRT will not treat these problems – it only effectively treats symptoms that are directly due to falling oestrogen levels – but it may indirectly make it easier to cope with stress. No one functions normally if they are tired and depressed. If it is just because night sweats frequently prevent a good night's sleep, HRT might be the answer.

The choice between the different types and ways of taking HRT is enormous, and the development of new treatments constantly increases the options. Many women do not need treatment at all. Even if you do, HRT is only one of many options available. The first regimen you try may not be the right one for you, so it is always worth trying a different type before you give up HRT altogether. Some people prefer the doctor to make the decisions for them. However, I hope this book will help you realize that you *can*, and should, play a part in that decision.

2

From Ancient Egypt to the Twenty-First Century

With all the recent interest in post-menopausal oestrogen deficiency and HRT you would be forgiven for thinking that the menopause is a modern 'disease'. But even the early philosophers and scientists were trying to unravel the mystery of why women stop menstruating, while men remain fertile until they die.

The first known references to the menopause date back to pre-biblical times; written accounts from ancient Egypt describe attempts at treatment, although in those days it was unlikely that many women lived long enough to reach the menopause.

Doctors living in medieval times thought that the menopause was caused by tumours growing inside the affected woman. A couple of centuries later the generally held belief was that the menstrual blood became stuck inside the body. This trapped blood was considered to be responsible for all the menopausal symptoms. Draining the blood out was an obvious answer, and the suggested cure was to apply leeches to the cervix.

The medical literature of the late eighteenth century refers to the menopause as a 'tragedy' and 'catastrophic attack'. Post-menopausal women were described as 'cow-like' or 'dull and unattractive'.

By the mid-nineteenth century doctors believed that during the menopause, the normal menstrual blood was expelled from the body as haemorrhages or hot flushes. After the menopause, the blood that was no longer expelled turned to fat instead.

At the turn of the twentieth century, the menopause was blamed for many physical and psychological diseases: tuberculosis, diabetes, depression, hysteria and insanity. If a woman suffered menopausal symptoms, it was all her own fault. This reflected the attitude of a male-dominated society at a time when women were starting to rebel against centuries of servitude. Support for the suffragette movement was cited as a cause of severe menopausal symptoms; indeed, any woman who was too highly educated, indulged in an undue amount of sex, or showed insufficient devotion to her husband or children, was bound to suffer.

The recommended treatment followed similar misconceptions. Women were supposed to avoid any sexual excitement at the menopause, since it might attract blood to the brain; if menstrual blood did manage to enter the brain, it would trigger mental symptoms, hot flushes, and perspiration.

Fortunately, the picture of the menopause was not always so gloomy. Some doctors had a more enlightened approach; they saw the menopause as the 'Indian Summer' of a woman's life – a time of extra energy, optimism, and even of physical beauty.

The development of HRT

Endless different remedies were suggested for menopausal symptoms. These ranged from herbs, purgatives, taking the waters and letting blood, to treatment with toxic metals such as lead.

Eventually the symptoms were linked to the cessation of ovarian function. This led to the first therapeutic trials to assess a treatment, reported in 1896. The therapies prescribed were extremely unpleasant; the choice was between: urine from pregnant women, fresh ovarian juice, extracts of ovaries and placentas, or powdered ovaries made up as tablets to be taken by mouth or implanted in the skin.

The active ingredient of these treatments remained a mystery for another quarter of a century. Edward Doisy, an American biochemist, was the first to identify the hormone oestrogen; in 1923, he detected this hormone in the urine of pregnant women. Soon after, in 1929, Edgar Allen discovered the second female sex hormone, progesterone. But even though the sex hormones had been identified, they could not easily be used as a treatment. The digestive juices inactivated the natural hormones when taken by mouth; the only effective method was to give them by injection.

The breakthrough came in the 1940s: scientists produced synthetic versions of the natural hormones, that in tablet form were sufficiently potent to withstand the digestive process. Premarin was also developed, a natural oestrogen that could be taken orally; it is still widely used today. Hormone replacement therapy had arrived.

Initially there was a great deal of uncertainty about the risks and benefits of HRT. Doctors already knew that it successfully treated the hot flushes and night sweats, but in 1940 researchers noted that women who had their ovaries removed subsequently had a greater risk of osteoporosis. Since the ovaries produce oestrogen, doctors reasoned that the most likely explanation was oestrogen deficiency.

When this finding was reported in the medical press, the number of prescriptions for oestrogen treatment dramatically increased.

The oral contraceptive pill was the next advance. The early pill combined high doses of synthetic oestrogen with a second hormone, progesterone. Although synthetic forms of progesterone had been developed in the 1950s by Djerassi and his colleagues, the pill did not become available in the USA until June 1960.

In 1961 came the first report linking the oral contraceptive pill with thrombosis. Research showed that the pill increased the risk of death from heart disease and stroke. Doctors believed that HRT would have the same effect, and prescriptions for HRT fell.

The tide turned again a few years later. New research suggested that the natural oestrogens used in HRT actually *protected* against heart disease. This difference between the effects of the oral contraceptive pill and HRT was explained by the fact that the pill contains high doses of synthetic oestrogen, necessary to prevent ovulation and act as a contraceptive. In contrast, HRT uses naturally occurring oestrogens at doses that are lower than the peak levels a woman will produce during her normal menstrual cycle; it has no contraceptive action.

HRT hit the headlines in 1966 with the publication of Robert Wilson's book *Feminine Forever*. This instant best-seller was the first book on the subject written specifically for the general public. It considerably heightened women's awareness that they did not have to suffer the menopause.

In the early 1970s clinics were set up especially for the study and treatment of the menopause. As interest grew, a group of doctors founded the International Menopause Society. A new medical journal, *Maturitas*, was launched and is still running, providing a forum for the publication of research findings.

It was not long before there were more scares about the safety of oestrogen replacement. Doctors noticed that the incidence of cancer of the uterus was increasing. A publication in 1975 reported the link between this cancer and oestrogen replacement therapy. It was also found that taking progestogen, a synthetic version of the hormone progesterone, prevented the development of cancer. Women with a uterus were advised to take progestogen, in addition to their oestrogen replacement.

But the damage had been done. Sensational newspaper headlines had reached patients and their doctors; women were wary of the possible long-term risks of hormone therapy, and its popularity again declined. This was in spite of the overwhelming evidence that the newer combination of oestrogen and progestogen was safe.

Then in 1981 the World Health Organization published a report in which the menopause was defined as an oestrogen deficiency disease. This 'disease' was considered to be an important risk factor, or even cause, of some of the chronic diseases associated with ageing: heart disease, strokes and osteoporosis.

Although many doctors agree with this concept, it is not a view held by everyone. Some doctors argue that although levels of oestrogen in menopausal women are lower than that necessary for reproductive function, many women produce sufficient oestrogen to maintain body tissues without the need for HRT. A few doctors even view the menopause as protective – protecting from unwanted pregnancy, or the risk of the genetic conditions, such as Down's syndrome, that are more common in children of older mothers.

Women themselves may consider the menopause to be a positive life event – relief from recurrent pre-menstrual symptoms, painful or heavy periods, and freedom from contraception can be a blessing. The menopause does not always have to be viewed with trepidation.

However, there is no doubt that for many women the use of hormone replacement therapy is associated with particular advantages. Nevertheless, like any drug, there are inherent risks from the treatment itself; any benefits need to be balanced against the possible risks, before the most suitable therapy can be chosen.

Many different drugs have been developed to treat the symptoms of the menopause, and to prevent the long-term complications of oestrogen withdrawal. Recent studies have confirmed the benefits of HRT on osteoporosis, which must be weighed against the slight increased risk of breast cancer. However, a question mark hangs over the effect of HRT on heart disease and stroke as certain types of HRT have been implicated in increased risk. This finding is in contrast with the expected actions of oestrogen on the body. Therefore it is likely that this risk may be relevant only to the type of HRT used in those studies and not to HRT in general. So research continues in an effort to find the safest, most effective form of treatment, which has the fewest side-effects. Naturally occurring oestrogens have superseded the synthetic oestrogens originally used in the 1940s, and more stable forms of natural progesterone are slowly replacing the synthetic progestogens. Patches, gels, nasal sprays, vaginal rings and implants are effective alternatives to pills. Each development gets closer to the goal – a treatment that can not only truly mimic the natural system but be even better.

3

From Menarche to Menopause

This chapter is for those of you interested in understanding the hormones involved in the menstrual cycle and the effects they have on the rest of the body. The events in a woman's reproductive life are covered, from the first menstrual period (menarche) to the last (the menopause). If you are not technically minded, you might find this chapter a little complicated. It is not essential to the basic understanding of HRT but if you have an idea of some of the ways that hormones work, you will realize the complexity of replacing the natural hormones with drugs.

The reproductive organs

Three main organs in the body are responsible for the control of the menstrual cycle: the hypothalamus, the pituitary gland and the ovaries.

The hypothalamus

The hypothalamus is the master gland of the body, the conductor of the hormonal orchestra. It sits at the base of the brain, just above the pituitary gland. The hypothalamus controls many of the body's functions – it regulates temperature, appetite, sleep, thirst, emotion and sexual behaviour. Diseases of the hypothalamus can have strange effects on eating behaviour: stimulating one part of the gland makes you hungry, stimulating another part makes you feel full. If a different part of the hypothalamus is damaged, you might feel permanently sleepy or thirsty.

The hypothalamus is also responsible for the various body rhythms, including the menstrual cycle. It produces at least seven different hormones, which control the pituitary gland.

The pituitary gland

The pituitary gland hangs down like a berry, under the brain. Under the control of the hypothalamic hormones, the pituitary secretes at least ten different hormones, two of which stimulate the ovaries. These are called the gonadotrophic hormones.

- *Follicle stimulating hormone* (FSH) controls the formation of eggs by the ovaries.
- *Luteinizing hormone* (LH) controls the production of sex hormones by the ovaries.

The ovaries

The ovaries are the most important female sex organs. A woman has two ovaries, one on each side of the uterus. In addition to containing the eggs, they produce the female sex hormones, oestrogen and progesterone.

When a girl is born her ovaries contain all the eggs she needs for the total of 400 to 500 times that she will ovulate from menarche to menopause. In contrast, men continue to make new sperm throughout their lives, until they die.

Twenty weeks after a baby girl is conceived, her developing ovaries contain 6–7 million immature eggs, called follicles. From this peak level, the number of follicles steadily decreases; by the time she is born, about 2 million remain; at puberty there are only 300,000.

During the reproductive years, numerous follicles start to develop during each menstrual cycle. Usually only one egg matures and is released from the ovary; the remaining eggs fail to develop properly and die. With this continuing decline, a mere few thousand eggs are left by the time of the menopause.

Puberty and the onset of menstruation

Adolescence, or puberty, is the time of sexual maturity. Strictly defined, it is the time when the sex organs have developed to the point where reproduction is possible. The ovaries start forming fertile eggs and produce the hormones that transform the shape of the body from a child to that of a woman.

Puberty lasts about two to four years, usually starting between the ages of 8 and 14. Delayed puberty – older than 17 in girls – is sometimes due to a shortage of the pituitary hormones. In rare cases, the hormonal changes triggering puberty start too early; precocious puberty has been recorded in a toddler who started menstruating at the age of 17 months!

Menarche

During the transition from child to woman, the levels of oestrogen in the body slowly rise. A sharp rise during the early teens triggers the menarche – the first menstrual period.

In the late nineteenth century the typical age at menarche was between 16 and 17 years. In developed countries this age has fallen over the centuries, probably because of higher living standards and improved nutrition; a recent ten-year study of middle-class American girls found that the average age at menarche was about 13, but varied from just over the age of 9 to over 17. In addition to health and nutrition, exposure to light, psychological factors and even geographic location affect the age at menarche: girls who live near to the equator, at lower altitudes or in towns are younger at their first period than those living at more northern latitudes, higher altitudes or in the country.

The control of puberty

No one is sure what controls the onset of puberty, but the hypothalamus seems to play a major part; some unknown mechanism triggers the hypothalamus to start producing the hormones that stimulate the ovaries and reproductive organs.

Slightly overweight girls start their periods earlier than girls of normal weight. This has led some doctors to suggest that reaching a critical body weight is the trigger for puberty. Others believe that the changes in the amount of body fat – increasing from 16 per cent in childhood to the adult female average of 23 per cent – is probably more important. But there is a great deal of individual variation. Genetic factors are involved as mothers, daughters and sisters are often of a similar age at their first period.

For a year or two after puberty, the body tries to adjust to the altered system of hormones. These changes upset the fine balance that exists, causing the typical adolescent problems – acne is common due to the sudden activity in the grease glands of the skin.

The menstrual cycle

The interaction between all the hormones involved is highly complex and the normal function of the menstrual cycle is one of the most remarkable events in human biology.

Every month after puberty, a single follicle matures and is released from the ovary. The lining of the uterus thickens in preparation for a possible pregnancy, providing a bed for the fertilized egg. If the egg is not fertilized, the uterus sheds its lining – the monthly 'period'. As soon as the bleeding is over, the lining regenerates, and the cycle starts again.

The average menstrual cycle takes 28 days – counted from the first day of one menstrual period to the start of the next – but the length is notoriously variable. The cycle can be divided into three stages: the follicular phase, ovulation, and the luteal phase. The first day of bleeding counts as day one of the cycle.

The follicular phase

The follicular phase is the first part of the cycle. Each follicle in the ovaries contains an immature egg. At the start of each cycle, hormones from the hypothalamus stimulate the pituitary gland to secrete *follicle stimulating hormone*. This stimulates the ovaries, and five to twenty follicles rapidly start to grow. By about day six of the cycle, a single follicle in one of the ovaries grows faster while the others regress.

The developing follicles produce the hormone *oestrogen* which instructs the pituitary gland to reduce the secretion of follicle stimulating hormone. As the cycle continues, oestrogen levels rise and eventually trigger the release of *luteinizing hormone* from the pituitary gland. *Ovulation* takes place as a surge of luteinizing hormone causes the follicle to rupture, releasing the mature egg into the abdomen. The egg is picked up by the finger-like ends of the fallopian tubes, and carried along towards the uterus.

The luteal phase

The luteal phase is the time between ovulation and menstruation. It consistently lasts close to 14 days. Under the control of luteinizing hormone, the empty follicle transforms itself into the *corpus luteum*. This 'yellow body' takes its name from the fatty yellowish cells that fill its cavity. The corpus luteum produces both oestrogen and progesterone. High levels of these two hormones cause the production of follicle stimulating hormone and luteinizing hormone to fall.

Meanwhile, the egg has travelled along the fallopian tubes towards the uterus. For pregnancy to take place, the egg must be fertilized by sperm within 12 to 24 hours of ovulation. If there is no pregnancy, the corpus luteum rapidly degenerates, nine to eleven days after ovulation. When the corpus luteum dies, the levels of oestrogen and progesterone fall. The newly formed lining of the uterus has lost its hormonal support, and breaks down. The cycle ends as the menstrual flow starts.

In contrast, if pregnancy does occur, the corpus luteum enlarges, secreting increased amounts of oestrogen and progesterone, necessary to maintain the pregnancy.

Menstruation

It has been said that 'menstruation is the womb weeping for its lost child'. The flow usually lasts between four and six days, but can range from two to eight days. Most of the blood is lost during the first three days of the period. The average total blood loss is about 30 ml, but this varies considerably between women.

The interval between ovulation and menstruation, the luteal phase, is nearly always two weeks. The interval between menstruation and the next ovulation, the follicular phase, varies from person to person and also from month to month in the same person. This means that a normal cycle can last anything from three to five weeks.

Throughout a woman's middle reproductive years cycles are regular, although they become more frequent with advancing age – mostly because the follicular phase shortens.

Women are most fertile when they are in their mid to late twenties. After this, fertility declines steadily until the menopause.

The menopause

Strictly defined, the menopause is the date of the last menstrual period. As women get older, the ovaries become less responsive to follicle stimulating hormone and luteinizing hormone. Between the ages of about 38 and 42, ovulation becomes less frequent. Fewer follicles remain in the ovaries and so less oestrogen is secreted. Eventually, too little oestrogen is produced to enable the lining of the uterus to thicken during each cycle. The final menstrual period occurs some time between the ages of 48 and 55. Premature menopause is when the menopause occurs under age 40.

The perimenopause

This is the name given to the phase from the start of symptoms of impending menopause – irregular periods, hot flushes, etc. – until 12 months after the last menstrual period.

The sex hormones

The ovaries produce large amounts of the female sex hormones, *oestrogen* and *progesterone*, as well as small amounts of the male hormones, *testosterone* and *androstenedione*. These male hormones, and a little oestrogen, are also secreted by another gland, the adrenal gland. There are two adrenal glands in the body, one on top of each of the kidneys.

Oestrogen

Oestrogen is a steroid hormone secreted by the developing follicles in the ovary before ovulation, by the corpus luteum after ovulation, and by the placenta during pregnancy. Smaller amounts are produced by the adrenal gland. Oestrogen is also formed in other tissues, particularly skin and fat. This can be an important source of oestrogen after the menopause.

During the normal menstrual cycle, most of the oestrogen comes from the ovary. The highest amounts can be measured just before ovulation. Another rise occurs in the middle of the second part of the cycle.

Actions of oestrogens

The female body

The changes in body shape at puberty are partly due to the presence of oestrogen and partly because women have low levels of testosterone. Breasts enlarge and nipples develop, the uterus and vagina grow and the voice stays high pitched. Women typically have narrow shoulders and broader hips, with a particular tendency to deposit fat on the hips and thighs. Under the control of oestrogen, women have less body hair and more scalp hair than men.

The menstrual cycle

Oestrogen is responsible for the development of the follicle. Together with progesterone, it stimulates the lining of the uterus to thicken. It also increases the lubricating mucous produced by glands in the cervix.

The cardiovascular system

Women have fewer heart attacks than men of a similar age – a difference which is particularly marked before the menopause. This seems to be due to the significant cholesterol-lowering action of oestrogen.

The skeleton

Oestrogen stops the growth of long bones (arms and legs): hence girls are usually shorter than boys. It is also important for keeping bones strong and healthy; the low levels of oestrogen after the menopause can lead to osteoporosis. This condition, often called 'brittle bones', increases the risk of fractures. The most common fractures affect the hip joint, the wrist and the spine. This can result in the condition known as 'the Dowager's hump'.

Progesterone

Progesterone is a steroid hormone secreted mostly by the corpus luteum in the ovary, during the second part of the menstrual cycle. It is known as the pregnancy hormone, stimulating the uterus already primed by oestrogen, in preparation for a possible pregnancy.

Actions of progesterone

The female body

Besides the changes in the uterus, progesterone is responsible for the development and multiplication of the glands in the breast. In the luteal phase of the menstrual cycle, high levels of progesterone cause the body temperature to rise slightly. This temperature change is sometimes used as an indicator of ovulation.

The menstrual cycle

Under the control of progesterone, the lining of the uterus develops glands during the luteal phase of the menstrual cycle. The cervical mucous thickens and becomes more acid. The muscle of the uterus relaxes and a much greater stimulus is needed to make it contract compared to during the follicular phase.

The sudden fall in the level of progesterone at the end of the cycle causes the menstrual bleed.

Other effects

Progesterone has been linked to the symptoms of pre-menstrual tension – weight gain, skin problems, irritability, painful breasts and fluid retention.

Testosterone and androstenedione

Men and women both make differing amounts of the same male and female sex hormones: levels of male hormones in women are about one tenth the amount measured in men.

After the menopause the ovary shrivels and secretes less oestrogen but the part of the ovary that produces the male hormones remains active. Levels of male hormones are raised for a few years following the menopause but eventually even this section of the ovary stops functioning.

Actions of male hormones
They are responsible for the growth of pubic and underarm hair. They do have other roles in the normal female but these are not entirely clear.

Summary

- In women, the most important hormones are oestrogen and progesterone.
- These are secreted by the ovaries, in varying amounts throughout the menstrual cycle.
- Oestrogen rises in the first part of the menstrual cycle and peaks at ovulation, when the egg is released from the ovary. Levels then fall but there is a second, more sustained rise in the second phase of the cycle, finally dropping again before menstruation.
- Progesterone levels are low in the first part of the cycle, and rise following ovulation. They also drop before menstruation.
- Two glands in the brain, the hypothalamus and the pituitary, control the production of hormones by the ovaries.
- None of these hormones acts in isolation and the result is an extremely complex system of control. Because of this, HRT cannot restore the pre-menopausal hormonal cycles.

4

The Climacteric

This chapter explains the symptoms that result from the hormonal changes leading up to, and beyond, the menopause. The following chapters explain the effects of HRT – the beneficial as well as the unwanted – and the different methods on offer. Alternatives to HRT are discussed in a later chapter.

The 'climacteric' is the medical term for all the hormonal changes that take place leading up to and following the menopause, marking the transition from the fertile to the non-fertile state. The age at the menopause has remained remarkably consistent over the centuries: today, the average age is just under 51, the same as shown in records from medieval times.

One major reason why the menopause has only recently received so much attention is that historically few women reached the age of 51 – only about 28 per cent of medieval women lived to experience the menopause, and fewer than 5 per cent survived to the age of 75. Today, 95 per cent of women living in developed countries reach the menopause, and the average life expectancy is now 83. So the menopause is a modern problem – nowadays most women are post-menopausal for a third of their life.

For many years, researchers have thought that no other primate living in its natural environment experienced the menopause. Old female rats and mice have long intervals without ovulating, but do not seem to have a menopause as such. The reason for this is unclear, but it seems likely that differences in life expectancy play a part: if the animals are kept in captivity, they live longer than in the wild. In this environment, some of them *do* experience a natural post-reproductive phase, although only one species, a particular strain of mouse, appears to have a true menopause.

The final menstrual period is the outward indication of the numerous internal changes that signal the 'change of life'.

These climacteric changes span many years, beginning around the age of 40, and end twenty to thirty years later when the reproductive organs start to fail.

For many women the first sign is a change in the pattern of menstruation: in the two to eight years before the final period, the cycles become irregular – the number of days between each period may vary, and the flow becomes heavier or more scanty. Eventually the periods stop altogether. Many of these cycles are anovulatory: that is, the egg fails to develop that month so there is no ovulation. Because of this the ovaries do not produce progesterone in the second part of that cycle; oestrogen continues to stimulate the lining of the uterus without the tempering effects of progesterone. These abnormal hormonal patterns can cause erratic bleeding, although the periods may still be at fairly regular intervals. In addition to these changes, the ovaries contain fewer follicles and are less able to produce oestrogen. Levels of oestrogen fluctuate, resulting in all the menopausal symptoms.

The menopause

The menopause is the medical term for the end of the monthly periods. It is the result of all the hormonal changes culminating in the cessation of the reproductive function of the ovaries.

Obviously, you cannot tell if the period you had last week is the final one, and since periods are often irregular around the time of the menopause, you may not have a period for two or three months. As a general rule, doctors consider that a woman has reached the menopause if she is over 45 and has not had a period for at least six months.

The menopause usually occurs between the ages of 48 and 55. About 1 per cent of women experience the menopause before the age of 40. It is not just hormonal changes that affect the age at the menopause: in a similar way to menarche, the menopause is affected by environmental differences – women who are heavy smokers or live at high altitudes tend to have an earlier menopause.

The symptoms can be disturbing, especially when they start much earlier than expected:

At the age of 43 I went to my GP complaining of night sweats, hot flushes, general tiredness, confusion, etc. I also had the sensation that my muscles, in particular my bladder muscles, weren't working properly at certain times of the menstrual month. I was also extremely tired, irritable and depressed. My periods became irregular and the tension would go on for weeks. Relief would

23

come for a few days with my period and then I would go off again on the downslide. I thought there was something wrong with my thyroid gland. The doctor thought it might be an early meno-pause, so he took some blood to check my hormone levels. I was shocked when the results confirmed that I was menopausal.

Hysterectomy and the menopause

If you have had a hysterectomy, especially if you were at a young age, you are one of a group that can particularly benefit from HRT.

Unless the ovaries are diseased or damaged in some way, usually only the uterus is removed at operation. The ovaries remain and function as before: the hormonal changes of the menstrual cycle take place each month, as normal, although without a uterus, there is no monthly bleed.

In the same way as at the natural menopause, symptoms start when the ovaries fail. This may be some years after the hysterec-tomy. However, there is some evidence that even if the ovaries are not removed, the operation itself may advance the natural meno-pause by about four years. In this instance, doctors recommend that HRT is taken at least until the age of 50, the average age at the menopause, although obviously it can be continued for longer if desired.

Occasionally the ovaries are removed as well as the uterus – a 'total' hysterectomy. This creates an artificial menopause and menopausal symptoms will start immediately. To combat this, many doctors prescribe HRT straight after the operation.

The reasons why you should consider HRT following a hysterec-tomy or an early menopause are discussed in the next chapter.

Oestrogen

The hormone, or rather the lack of it, that is responsible for many of the physical changes during the climacteric, is oestrogen. Many tissues throughout the body are sensitive to oestrogen:

- genital organs (vagina, vulva and uterus);
- urinary organs (bladder and urethra);
- brain;
- breasts;

- skin;
- hair;
- muscles;
- blood vessels;
- bones.

The levels of oestrogen in the body normally start to fall from about the age of 35. This decline speeds up at the menopause as there are fewer follicles remaining in the ovary. The number of follicles may be important for triggering the menopause, but some doctors believe that the menopause might be due to 'pre-programming' of the brain, probably the hypothalamus.

Whatever the mechanism, the follicles containing the eggs become less sensitive to the effects of the pituitary hormones, follicle stimulating hormone (FSH) and luteinizing hormone (LH).

Even if the follicles do manage to grow, they produce less oestrogen than their predecessors. As the levels of oestrogen fall, the pituitary gland produces more follicle stimulating hormone, in an attempt to coerce the follicle to develop and secrete more oestrogen. This is a useful test for the menopause; a blood test will show high levels of follicle stimulating hormone. But for most women this test is unnecessary, as the symptoms of irregular periods, hot flushes and night sweats are sufficient evidence.

Eventually, the follicles fail to respond to the pituitary hormones, and the remaining eggs cannot mature. Some doctors maintain that this may be nature's way of preventing genetic abnormalities: the eggs left in the ovaries at the menopause are not as healthy as the ones that matured in the early reproductive years. Many appear defective, containing a higher number of abnormal genes in the chromosomes. This is why women who become pregnant in their late forties have a much higher risk of having a baby with Down's syndrome (mongolism) than younger women.

Oestrogen after the menopause
The body produces three different types of oestrogen:

- oestradiol;
- oestriol;
- oestrone.

Oestradiol is the most potent and, before the menopause, the most abundant of the oestrogens. After the menopause the levels of oestradiol fall, and the regular pattern of changes that occurred over the menstrual cycle ceases. Levels of the other two oestrogens, oestrone and oestriol, do not change dramatically, remaining similar to the early stage of the normal menstrual cycle.

Not every woman suffers the effects of oestrogen deficiency. Even though the ovaries stop producing oestrogen after the menopause, a significant amount may still be measured in the bloodstream. This is because production of the male hormone, androstenedione, increases and is converted to oestrogen.

Before the menopause, most of the male hormones come from the adrenal gland, and only a small amount is secreted by the ovaries. After the menopause, most of the ovarian tissue stops responding to the increasing concentrations of follicle stimulating hormone and luteinizing hormone. However, the part of the ovary that secretes the male hormones *does* respond; production of testosterone and androstenedione continues for several years after the oestrogen-secreting part of the ovary has withered.

The amount of androstenedione that is converted to oestrogen varies from one woman to another but there may be enough to prevent the loss of tissue from the breasts and vagina. Fat women have higher post-menopausal levels of oestrogen than thinner women: androstenedione is converted to oestrogen in fat cells.

However, the oestrogen produced after the menopause differs in several ways from oestrogen produced before the menopause:

- Post-menopausal oestrogen is primarily oestrone, whereas oestradiol from the ovaries is the principal oestrogen in pre-menopausal women.
- Post-menopausal oestrone secretion is at a constant level of production. This is in contrast to oestradiol secretion by pre-menopausal women, which characteristically rises and falls throughout the menstrual cycle with a peak immediately before the egg is released from the ovary.

Eventually, several years after the menopause, the ovaries stop functioning completely and oestrogen levels fall further.

26

Irregular bleeding

Any unusual bleeding both before and after the menopause, on or off hormone replacement therapy, should be reported to your doctor. In the majority of cases, the cause is not serious – fibroids, endometriosis or polyps. But there is always the potential risk of a more sinister problem, such as cancer. However slight this risk is, early treatment means a greater chance of full recovery.

Before the menopause:
Irregular bleeding is most often due to a failure to ovulate: if no egg is released during the cycle, the effects of oestrogen are then 'unopposed' by progesterone, and the periods become erratic.

Hormonal changes are not the only cause of irregular periods; all the following can affect the menstrual cycle:

* emotion;
* changes in the environment;
* illness;
* changes in body weight: research shows that rapid weight loss and dieting too strictly can shorten the menstrual cycle;
* disease: polyps, cervical erosions, or other non-cancerous conditions of the vagina, cervix or uterus. Rarely, cancer.

Irregular bleeding after the menopause
This can be caused by a number of things.

* Bleeding is a side-effect of hormone replacement therapy.
* A few women produce large amounts of androstenedione, which is converted to oestrogen. These unusually high levels of oestrogen can cause post-menopausal bleeding.
* Non-cancerous disease of the vagina, cervix or uterus. It may rarely be an early sign of cancer of the uterus.

The menopause syndrome

Oestrogen withdrawal results in a variety of symptoms. The most obvious symptoms, the hot flushes and night sweats, only last a few years at most, until the levels of oestrogen stabilize at lower levels. However, the levels of oestrogen do not necessarily equate to the degree and severity of symptoms and fluctuating oestrogen levels seem more important than a persistently low level. The symptoms can be extremely disturbing, especially following an early menopause. More recently, long-term health problems have been recognized as a consequence of oestrogen deficiency, in particular osteoporosis and heart disease.

Menopausal symptoms

Hot flushes and night sweats

Hot flushes are the commonest symptom of the climacteric; at least 60 per cent of women notice them within three months of a natural or artificial menopause. They usually abate after a few months, but in 25 per cent of women they can persist for up to five years.

Surprisingly, even men occasionally experience flushes; they sometimes occur in men treated for cancer of the prostate gland.

For some women, a flush means nothing more than an occasional sense of warmth lasting from 30 seconds up to five minutes at the most. Others notice reddening of the skin over their chests, rising up to the neck and face, accompanied by a feeling of intense heat. This can be followed by profuse perspiration, particularly at night. Weakness, dizziness and feeling faint are other common symptoms. Flushes can occur frequently during the day, but night sweats are most troublesome, particularly since they disrupt sleep, leading to tiredness and irritability the following day. A few unlucky women experience hourly waves of heat, drenching sweats, heart racing and a feeling of anxiety:

> I started my menopause at the age of 51. The hot flushes and night sweats started a year later. I would have up to 30 hot flushes in a day – sometimes they seemed to last all day. The night sweats weren't so frequent, but enough to wake me up; often I would have to change my nightdress because I was so drenched.

Some women can sense that a flush is beginning, with warning palpitations or a headache. Doctors do not understand the exact mechanism of the hot flush: it appears to be a response to a sudden, but transient, downward setting of the body's thermostat, located in the hypothalamus. This temporary alteration of the central temperature setting point causes the sensation of intense heat. In turn, this

28

activates heat loss responses: flushing, sweating and feeling the need to remove clothing. At the same time, the hypothalamus secretes *gonadotrophin releasing hormone* (GnRH) which stimulates a surge of luteinizing hormone (LH) from the pituitary gland. For a long time, doctors thought that this was the trigger of the flushes, but it seems to be an associated event, not the cause.

The removal of both ovaries creates an artificial menopause, and the abrupt drop in oestrogen causes hot flushes immediately following the operation, relieved by oestrogen therapy. Women born with abnormal ovaries that cannot produce oestrogen have very low levels of oestrogen in their body, but they do not suffer from hot flushes. However, if they are given oestrogen therapy, they experience all the menopausal symptoms when the oestrogen therapy is stopped. This shows that the change in the levels of oestrogen, from high to low, is the important factor, which is why the hot flushes stop when the oestrogen levels settle at low levels a few years after the menopause.

Difficulty sleeping

Insomnia can result from emotional problems, which may or may not be secondary to oestrogen withdrawal. More commonly interrupted sleep is due to constantly waking with the night sweats.

Headaches

In one study of women with migraine attending a menopause clinic, nearly 40 per cent said that their migraine had deteriorated during the climacteric.

Until puberty, boys and girls are equally likely to have migraine. After puberty, three times as many women suffer from migraine as men. This is most likely a hormonal effect, particularly since migraine is affected by the various hormonal events throughout a woman's life.

Some women notice a link between their migraines and menstrual periods. 'Menstrual migraine' is the term given to attacks that start within a couple of days before or after the first day of menstruation.

Doctors do not fully understand why such a relationship should develop at this stage of life, although a few women do notice a link with their periods when they are younger. The hypothalamus is probably involved; besides its function controlling the menstrual cycle, it is also implicated in migraine.

For most women, the attacks subside after the menopause, but this is not always the case; about 10 per cent of women continue to have migraine.

Non-migraine headaches are also more common at the time of the menopause. The causes of these are numerous: the changing hormonal environment may be partly responsible and HRT can both aggravate or relieve headaches. Stress, lack of sleep and depression can all result in a tension headache. Skeletal problems and neck pain become more of a problem with advancing years and can lead to headaches besides triggering migraine.

Emotional symptoms

Depression

Most people have felt a bit low at some time in their lives. Often it is shortly after the death of a friend or relative; they get over it with time. Real depression is something quite different. Depressed people find it difficult to feel happy about anything or to show any emotional reaction. They wake in the early hours of the morning and find it impossible to get back to sleep. They lose weight because they cannot be bothered to eat properly. Depression is not something that can be 'shaken off' – often there does not seem any particular reason why the person should feel so down.

Women in their middle years have a high risk of depressive illness, but few studies have confirmed a link between depression and the menopause. If depression does occur, there has usually been a similar episode in the past.

Hormone replacement therapy is unlikely to treat depression effectively, unless the depression is secondary to other menopausal symptoms; if hot flushes and night sweats cause loss of sleep, itself resulting in depression, then HRT may be an effective therapy.

Other symptoms

Physical symptoms are only part of the changes during the climacteric. Psychological symptoms can include:

- anxiety;
- mood changes;
- irritability;
- forgetfulness;
- poor concentration;

- difficulty sleeping;
- tiredness and loss of energy.

Studies show that these symptoms increase in association with the menopause. However, other factors may also be important. The menopause occurs at a time of many other life stresses: the family may have grown up or left home, ending the role as a mother; retirement is approaching; parents are often in poor health, or die.

All these external factors have an effect, and psychological problems during the climacteric are only partly, if at all, due to oestrogen deficiency. Over-tiredness caused by frequent night sweats can be responsible for many of the psychological symptoms. But depression, anxiety, poor memory, feelings of inadequacy and loss of sexual drive, all depend on several additional factors: basic personality, the rate of change of the physical effects of ageing and severity of symptoms, and social situation.

But it is important to consider that these same life events can also have a positive effect. Retirement can mean the time to fulfil other ambitions, and children leaving home gives you the chance to be alone with your partner.

Sexual difficulties

Oestrogen deficiency does not directly affect libido, but relationships with partners have to survive additional stresses arising from the physical and psychological changes that affect a woman during the climacteric. However, many of these problems will have been building up over several years and the menopause only acts as a catalyst.

The physical changes that can tighten and dry the skin of the vagina, causing pain on intercourse, do not happen until several years after the menopause. Continued sexual activity can itself stimulate vaginal secretions, without the added stimulus of oestrogen replacement.

It is frequently stated that men and women lose interest in sex as they get older. One study of sexual activity in married women found a decline with age, paralleled by a decline in sexual intercourse with their partners. As sexual activity in single women remained unchanged, the researchers concluded that the decline in sexual activity between married women and their spouses was linked to other difficulties. Perhaps the marriage is not as happy as it was;

perhaps other external stresses or underlying depression are the root of the problem.

It is not uncommon to experience sexual difficulties, ranging from emotional problems – usually loss of interest – to physical problems, such as pain on intercourse. Sometimes your partner may feel angry and frustrated at your lack of interest, or simply be afraid of hurting you. Emotional problems often coexist with physical problems. Sexual difficulties are partnership problems so discuss them with your partner, asking your doctor for help if necessary.

Joint and muscle pain

Aching joints, particularly the hip joints, and pain in the lower back are frequent complaints. The ageing process also results in a steady loss of muscular strength. These changes are affected by many physical factors, including build and weight as well as physical fitness. The role of oestrogen is uncertain but studies have shown that taking HRT can ease joint pains and limit the natural decline in muscle power. Furthermore, there is some evidence that oestrogen, taken before there is evidence of joint disease, provides some protection against rheumatoid arthritis.

Eyes

Some eye complaints seemed linked to oestrogen withdrawal: a recent study in Austria showed that 35 per cent of women attending a clinic for treatment of their menopausal symptoms complained of deteriorating vision and dry, red eyes.

Skin

Sunlight and the general process of ageing are the real culprits responsible for wrinkles and patches of pigmentation (often called 'liver spots'). It is possible that the lack of oestrogen contributes to the general loss of elasticity and thinning of the skin and hair, but it is not the sole cause.

Some women experience a particularly unpleasant sensation of something 'crawling' under their skin, called formication. Although the cause is unknown, it does respond to HRT.

The reproductive tissues and the bladder

Over the years the breasts gradually become smaller and less firm. Of more importance to many women are the effects of oestrogen deficiency on the bladder and the genital tract. In contrast to hot flushes, these problems start several years after the menopause, at about the age of 60.

The vulva

This is the term given to the external female genitalia that surround the entrance to the vagina. The skin of the vulva thins and can become very chapped and sore, although these changes are not usually seen until many years after the menopause.

The vagina

Like the other tissues, the lining of the vagina may eventually become thin and inflamed, making intercourse painful. The blood flow to the vagina also decreases, and the skin becomes dry as the glands produce less of the lubricating secretions. Continued sexual activity seems to prevent some of these changes, even without oestrogen replacement – pleasurable emotions increase the blood flow, and lubrication increases as the glands are stimulated.

The uterus

With advancing years the uterus shrinks and the supporting tissues lose their strength and elasticity. Eventually the uterus may 'prolapse' or slip down, sometimes appearing as a painless lump at the entrance to the vagina. This is more noticeable when standing or coughing and usually disappears on lying down. In the same way, the rectum and bladder can also prolapse.

Women who have had children are more likely to have a prolapsed uterus, as pregnancy weakens many of the supporting ligaments and muscles, but it occasionally affects women who have not been pregnant. Obese women are also at greater risk.

Lack of oestrogen may be an additional factor in the loss of muscle tone but HRT will not prevent prolapse of the uterus. An operation can help treat prolapse, by tightening up the supporting structures. Otherwise, a plastic ring can be inserted into the vagina to prevent the vaginal walls collapsing.

The bladder

The lining of the bladder thins, becomes drier, is more prone to infections and irritations, and loses some of its muscle tone. This leads to loss of control, causing the feeling of a frequent need to urinate. All too often this happens during the night, interrupting sleep that is already disturbed by night sweats.

Stress incontinence is a further problem – coughing, sneezing, even laughing can lead to slight leaking of the bladder. Incontinence is very common – it is one of the leading reasons for institutionalization of the elderly, second only to dementia.

The urethra, the duct by which urine passes from the bladder, can become inflamed, making it painful to urinate. Occasionally the urethra becomes infected, needing treatment with antibiotics.

Breast disease

Around the time of the menopause, painful breasts and cysts are common. Fortunately, in most cases the symptoms are short-lived, until the hormonal changes settle down.

After the menopause, these harmless lumps and cysts are less common. In contrast, the incidence of breast cancer increases steadily with age, so any lumps should always be checked by the doctor.

Long-term effects of the menopause

Strokes and heart disease

In many Western countries, cerebrovascular diseases, which include heart disease and stroke, are the major cause of death: in the United States, nearly 53 per cent of all deaths occurring in women over the age of 50 are due to cerebrovascular disease. This compares to 4 per cent of deaths from breast cancer, 18 per cent from all other cancers, and 2 per cent from accidents and suicides, within the same age group.

Women are less likely to suffer from heart disease than men of the same age, but more women than men die from heart disease overall. This apparent contradiction can be explained by the fact that, on average, women develop heart disease about seven to eight years later than men.

Oestrogens have been associated with the low rate of heart disease in pre-menopausal women, compared to men of the same age, yet the natural menopause does not cause an immediate increase in risk for heart disease. The ovarian production of oestrogen begins to decline from the age of 40, and the whole shutting-down process may take ten to fifteen years or more. Because of this, it is unlikely that any abrupt menopausal effect on cerebrovascular disease would be seen. This contrasts with the mortality rates for breast cancer, in which a menopausal effect is clearly evident.

34

However, the menopause does signal a period of increasing risk. There is also abundant support for the observation that women who have had both ovaries surgically removed have an increased risk of heart disease, as they lose the final years of oestrogen protection.

Nevertheless, lack of oestrogen is not the only factor linking heart disease and the menopause. The likelihood that any individual will have a heart attack depends on the number of 'risk' factors present; most of you will be aware that high blood pressure and high cholesterol levels increase your risk, especially if any close relatives have had heart attacks or strokes.

Three important risk factors for heart disease can themselves affect the timing of the menopause:

- age – two-thirds of women experience the menopause between 48 and 53 years;
- cigarette smoking – associated with an early menopause;
- obesity – associated with a later menopause.

Oestrogen and cholesterol

Studies show that cholesterol levels start to rise after the menopause as the cholesterol-lowering action of oestrogen is lost. High levels of cholesterol in the blood are associated with a greater risk of heart disease.

Special proteins carry cholesterol in the bloodstream: the two most important are *low density lipoproteins* (LDL) and *high density lipoproteins* (HDL). The low density lipoprotein carrier has been linked to the build-up of fatty deposits inside blood vessels. This can restrict the normal blood flow, resulting in heart attacks or strokes. In contrast, high density lipoproteins clean up the fatty deposits, protecting against heart disease.

The ratio of the two lipoproteins is important – people with the greatest risk of heart attacks have a high ratio; they have much more low density lipoprotein in the bloodstream than high density lipoprotein. Other factors, including male hormones and age, increase this ratio. Oestrogen decreases it.

Osteoporosis

Osteoarthritis is often confused with osteoporosis since both become more common with increasing age. The bony surfaces of a joint become worn with age, especially if the joint has been injured, causing pain and stiffness. An X-ray shows loss of the normal space between the bones, areas of hardening of bone – sclerosis – and small pieces of new bone growing on the surface of the joint. These changes are typical of osteoarthritis.

Osteoporosis is the name given to the thinning of bone. On an X-ray film, osteoporotic bone appears less dense than normal bone.

The strength of a bone is due to its structure of protein fibres and hard crystals of the mineral calcium phosphate. Reduced amounts of bone protein and calcium make the bone more fragile, increasing the risk of fractures, especially of the hips, wrists and spine. After the menopause, circulating oestrogen drops and the bones lose minerals faster than they gain them.

But oestrogen deficiency is not the sole cause of osteoporosis: long-term immobilization and ageing are other factors. There is also a racial difference – Caucasian and oriental women start losing bone earlier than African or Caribbean women. Women are more at risk of fractures than men – by the age of 60 about 7 per cent of women will have fractured a bone that has been weakened by osteoporosis. At 80 years, an estimated 25 per cent of women are affected. In contrast, about 3 per cent of 60-year-old men have had a fracture, and only 8 per cent by the age of 80.

The overall risk of fractures depends on three main factors:

- the peak amount of bone mass;
- the age at which bone loss begins;
- the subsequent rate at which the bone is lost.

All untreated women will, to some extent, lose bone mass after the menopause. It takes about ten to fifteen years before the results of this become apparent, but the loss is greatest in the first few years.

The wrists, hips and spine are the commonest parts of the body affected, and between the ages of 35 and 60 there is a ten-fold increase in Colles fractures, affecting the wrists. The risk of fractures of the hip is even greater: 80 per cent of hip fractures are directly linked with osteoporosis. Treatment causes further problems: surgery carries its own risks, and staying in bed after the operation increases the chance of blood clots in the legs and lungs, and chest infections. Getting up and about, under the care of a physiotherapist, as soon as possible after a major operation can minimize these problems. Unfortunately, long-term disability following hip operations, particularly affecting mobility, is quite common.

About one third of women over the age of 65 have a fracture of the spinal bones – the vertebrae – which literally collapse. This is the cause of the Dowager's hump and loss of height – an average of 2.5 inches in an untreated post-menopausal woman. Breathing, stomach and bladder problems may result, and the pressure of the collapsed bone on the nerves emerging from the spinal column leads to a great deal of pain.

Gravity, exercise and diet play a part – osteoporosis is a problem for astronauts as they lose the benefit of the earth's gravitational pull. For this reason, exercises that work against gravity, such as weight training, afford better protection against osteoporosis than non-gravitational exercises like swimming.

Many people in affluent societies have cut down their intake of dairy produce in an attempt to reduce their fat intake. But milk, butter and cheese are important sources of calcium – one explanation for the increasing number of fractures in elderly people is a low dietary calcium intake.

Fluoride, added to tap water in some countries, is a potent stimulator of bone formation but the large number of side-effects it produces limit its use in the prevention of fractures.

The sunshine vitamin, vitamin D – so named because sunlight stimulates the production of this vitamin in the skin – is important for the development and growth of healthy bones but has little effect on preventing fractures.

Oestrogen deficiency is the most important factor, particularly affecting the vertebral bones. It has a direct protective effect on bone besides aiding calcium absorption. Bone is a highly active material, and is constantly broken down and replaced – it does not bear any resemblance to the skeletons seen in museums. Two different types of cells are involved in the turnover of bone: *osteoblasts* build up bone and *osteoclasts* break it down. Oestrogen stimulates osteoblasts, which form new bone. Synthetic progesterone, usually combined with oestrogen as part of the HRT regime, also builds up bone mass.

Summary

- The climacteric spans the ten to twenty years of hormonal changes. The ovaries gradually become less responsive to the stimulating hormones from the pituitary gland, and secrete less oestrogen. This culminates in the menopause, the last menstrual period.

- The fluctuating levels of oestrogen produce the symptoms of the menopause – hot flushes, night sweats, difficulty sleeping, depression and palpitations, to name a few.
- Most of these symptoms only last for several months – a few years at the most – until the levels of oestrogen have stabilized at the lower level.
- Oestrogen deficiency is not the sole cause of the symptoms that a woman may experience during the climacteric. The effects of the numerous changes that take place depend on several variables: inherited factors, physical build, and the psychological ability to cope with the ageing process as well as the emotional impact of 'the change of life'. Each of these is as important as the amount and rate of oestrogen loss.
- More recently, the longer-term effects of the menopause have been recognized. Oestrogen deficiency is associated with an increasing risk of heart disease, strokes and fractures.

5
Why take HRT? The Plus Factors

The benefits of HRT are discussed in this chapter – how HRT relieves menopausal symptoms and its role in the prevention of osteoporosis. Prevention is important, as many women with osteoporosis do not have any symptoms: all too often the first sign is the external evidence of underlying disease – a broken wrist or hip. Therefore this chapter also includes sections on how to assess your own likelihood of developing osteoporosis.

Replacing the oestrogen

The aim of HRT is to replace the oestrogens that the ovaries no longer produce after the menopause. Oestrogen replacement cannot keep the ravages of age at bay; nevertheless, it can slow down the changes accelerated by the menopause:

> *I have felt much better since I've been on HRT – it definitely improves my skin and hair. I feel confident it will help keep my bones strong as I get older. It is also helpful enabling much easier sexual intercourse by keeping the area moist. I feel in much better general health, and now go swimming regularly. My family and friends say I look better too.*

The menopause itself is not a disease. Yet many doctors feel that its effects on the heart and bones, the reproductive organs, the bladder and skin, combine to produce a host of psychological and physical problems. Post-menopausal women face an increased risk of heart disease and strokes. Osteoporosis is responsible for a higher risk of fractures. These can all have fatal consequences.

Studies suggest that between 75 and 85 per cent of women experience troublesome menopausal symptoms, especially hot flushes and night sweats. Most are relatively mild and short-lived, though some can be severe and incapacitating. Although it is known that hormone replacement therapy effectively relieves many of these symptoms, it can be difficult for researchers to establish exactly how effective any treatment is. Some women respond to investigation of their symptoms – this means that a percentage of women will improve just by discussing their problems with the doctor.

Many doctors feel that every woman should be given the opportunity to take HRT. Some even see the menopause as an unnatural event, as it appears to be almost exclusively a human phenomenon. This is probably because our life expectancy has increased dramatically over the last century. In contrast, the life expectancy of animals living in their natural state has stayed much the same. However, recent work shows that some animals in captivity live longer than in the wild, and do appear to experience a menopause.

There are at least two important reasons why a woman might consider hormone replacement therapy.

- Short-term use, up to five years, relieves the hot flushes and night sweats as well as vaginal and bladder problems.
- Long-term therapy can reduce the risk of osteoporosis. Treatment should be continued life-long since bone density falls when HRT is stopped.

Hysterectomy and early menopause

A particular group of women who can benefit from HRT are those who have an early menopause. This may be a natural menopause, or the consequence of surgical removal of the ovaries. An early menopause can be triggered by a hysterectomy, even if the ovaries are not removed. Whatever the reason for an early menopause, the risk of heart disease and osteoporosis is increased, as the protection provided by oestrogen is lost at an earlier age than usual. Because of this, most doctors agree that these women should take HRT at least until they reach 51, the average age at menopause.

Symptom relief

Replacing the lost oestrogen treats many of the symptoms of the change. The effect can be quite dramatic, but do not expect any miracles.

The most common symptoms are hot flushes, night sweats and insomnia. During the months leading up to the menopause, irregular periods and loss of the normal hormonal balance result in erratic fluctuations in oestrogen levels. Some researchers suggest that the rate of change of oestrogen triggers the hot flushes. Others think that there is a critical range of oestrogen: if the level is within this range, hot flushes occur; above or below this level and they will not. This would explain why the hot flushes eventually stop of their own accord as oestrogen falls below the critical level. Similarly, HRT will raise the level of oestrogen above the critical range.

Unfortunately, oestrogen falls again when HRT is discontinued and some of the symptoms may return for a short time. These eventually cease when the oestrogen levels stabilize again, at a lower level, but can be prevented by slowly tapering the dose of oestrogen over several weeks or months.

Hot flushes and night sweats
HRT effectively stops the hot flushes; sometimes improvement is apparent within a few days of starting treatment. Usually the response is more gradual, continuing over the first three months of treatment.

Difficulty sleeping
HRT can help sleep, preventing the resultant drenching from night sweats. Better sleep helps relieve other symptoms – depression, irritability and poor concentration – which are often simply due to tiredness.

Difficulty getting to sleep is another problem of the menopause that can respond to HRT.

Headaches
HRT can both aggravate and improve migraine headaches; unfortunately there is no way of judging its effect. Some women find they are more prone to headaches when taking the course of progestogen or shortly after, during the withdrawal bleeding. Changing the dose or type of hormones, or switching to a different route of HRT, can solve the problem.

Sometimes HRT is just an additional trigger, so it is important to look for other underlying causes for the headaches.

Emotional symptoms
Oestrogen can act as a mental tonic: a link between low levels of oestrogen and low levels of beta-endorphins has been found – these are natural brain chemicals. Raising the levels of oestrogen seems to raise levels of these mood-enhancing chemicals.

Depression, forgetfulness and feelings of anxiety can result from sleepless nights. Treating hot flushes and night sweats with HRT helps to restore the normal sleep pattern and may, in turn, treat the depression.

But hormonal changes cannot take all the blame for depression and emotional upsets. Extra pressures and responsibilities – retirement, death of a close relative, etc. – often coincide with this stage of life, and menopausal symptoms can make it harder to cope. The menopause marks a woman's loss of fertility and youth; it may also increase her awareness of her own mortality and that of her friends and family. It is not always easy to adjust to these changes. In these cases, HRT is unlikely to make much difference; the only effective treatment is to resolve the underlying problems.

Sexual difficulties
The tissues of the vulva and the vagina are particularly sensitive to oestrogen. After the menopause these tissues can become thin and dry, making intercourse painful. Regular intercourse is thought to prevent this: sexual excitement moistens the walls of the vagina, and stimulates the glands in the vagina to secrete a lubricating fluid. If HRT is not necessary for any other reason, oestrogen creams can be used for a few weeks, and repeated when necessary. The cream is inserted into the vagina using a special applicator. Pessaries, vaginal tablets and a vaginal ring are also available.

Libido
Improving vaginal dryness with oestrogen treatment has been shown to restore sexual desire. Testosterone, the male hormone, is responsible for sex drive. Studies show that supplementing oestrogen replacement with testosterone can help to restore libido. Tibolone, a synthetic HRT, is also effective for libido.

Joint and muscle pain
HRT may improve pain affecting the joints of the hands, wrist, elbows and shoulders that occasionally starts around the menopause.

Eyes
The eyes are bathed in tears all the time and tears contain natural antibiotics to keep the eyes healthy. Some women make less tear fluid after the menopause, and their eyes become sore, dry and red.

Vision also deteriorates with age, although it is now thought that oestrogen deficiency also plays a part. A small study showed that women could focus better after just three months' treatment with HRT. They also produced a greater quantity of tears.

Skin
From about the age of 40 the skin rapidly starts to thin. This is mostly due to the ageing process, but HRT can help reduce the additional thinning caused by lack of oestrogen. Some indirect evidence suggests that HRT helps to maintain collagen, which forms the basic structure of skin. It also appears to protect against varicose ulcers.

Hair
Hair starts to thin after the menopause, but HRT can improve both its thickness and condition.

Urinary symptoms
Incontinence is a more common problem than many people realize. A study in Sweden found that 12 per cent of 50-year-old women and over 25 per cent of women in their eighties leak urine from their bladder. When 346 incontinent women took oestrogen therapy, there was a marked improvement in symptoms such as pain on passing water, or feeling the need to empty the bladder frequently, especially at night. They also had fewer problems with cystitis and vaginal infections.

Osteoporosis

An individual woman has a one in six chance of fracturing a bone during her life. By the age of 30, the bone mass has reached its peak; from that point on it gradually reduces with age. After the menopause, there is no more protection from oestrogen and the rate at which bone is lost suddenly increases.

Osteoporosis is a major risk factor for fractures. Fractures cause tremendous long-term problems of mobility: up to 50 per cent of women with a fractured hip become less mobile after the accident. You also lose your independence, needing to rely on other people to help you through simple daily tasks. The risk of death following hip fracture is significant, around 15 to 25 per cent six months after the injury.

Who is at risk of osteoporosis?

As for heart disease and strokes, charts of risk factors for osteoporosis can only give an indication of the risk within a specific population. They are of little value in assessing the risk of an individual, but a high number of risk factors does indicate a greater risk.

Risk factors for osteoporosis include:

- early menopause or 'total' hysterectomy (with surgical removal of the ovaries);
- a history of irregular periods or long gaps without menstruating (amenorrhoea);
- low body weight or history of anorexia nervosa;
- low dietary intake of calcium;
- lack of exercise;
- smoking;
- alcohol intake;
- racial origin;
- presence of certain diseases that lead to osteoporosis (e.g. thyrotoxicosis);
- long-term use of oral steroids, e.g. prednisolone;
- a blood relative who has osteoporosis;
- a fracture of the hip or wrist before the age of 65.

Hormones

An early menopause or long-standing amenorrhoea increases the risk of osteoporosis. In contrast, conditions that raise the levels of oestrogen – pregnancy, or taking the oral contraceptive pill – help build up a greater peak bone mass, and hence reduce the risk of osteoporosis.

Weight

Thin women, especially those who have had anorexia nervosa or bulimia, are more at risk of osteoporosis than fatter women. A low body weight is associated with lower levels of oestrogen and greater loss of bone. One way to assess your risk is to calculate your Body Mass Index. This can easily be calculated using the following formula:

Body Mass Index = weight (kg)/(height in metres)^2

This gives a simple numerical index. A woman's ideal BMI should be between 19 and 25. If it is below 19, you run a greater risk of osteoporosis.

Calcium

Calcium plays an important role: the amount of calcium in your diet when you were a child, particularly during the pubertal growth spurt, seems to determine the quantity of bone in your skeleton as an adult.

Exercise

If you exercised regularly as a child and in early adult life, you will have a greater bone mass than more sedentary individuals. Women are generally less physically active than men and take less exercise as they get older, so it is important to continue weight-bearing exercises such as walking and dancing, to protect against bone loss.

But you can take it too far. Some women athletes have very little fat on their bodies and their periods stop. This actually increases the risk of osteoporosis.

Smoking

Smoking harms the skeleton for three reasons:

- If you smoke heavily you are likely to have an earlier menopause – up to two to five years earlier than if you did not smoke.
- Smoking speeds up the turnover of oestrogen so there is less of it in the bloodstream.
- Smoking also appears to affect the formation of new bone.

Alcohol

Too much alcohol is also bad for bone, though no one seems sure exactly what level counts as 'too much'. Certainly, alcoholics are more likely to develop osteoporosis, although they usually also have a poor diet, with little calcium. However, some doctors have suggested that even modest social drinking is a potential cause of bone loss.

Race

Negroid women have a much denser skeleton than white women so are less likely to get osteoporosis than Caucasians or Asians. An early menopause, especially under the age of 40, is a high risk factor, as is having a mother or grandmother who lost height or developed a Dowager's hump. Chronic illness, particularly if you are confined to bed, also increases your risk.

Medical causes
Lack of oestrogen is not the only cause of osteoporosis. Certain medical conditions, such as an overactive thyroid and diabetes, are associated with osteoporosis.

Screening for osteoporosis

Obviously not every woman will suffer from osteoporosis, and even if you have severe osteoporosis it does not necessarily mean that your bones will fracture. Screening would be a useful way to identify those at risk. Unfortunately, screening tests are not widely available at present. The only reliable test currently available is bone density measurement, which is expensive. Several screening tools are being researched, including the use of ultrasound. These techniques measure bone mass more accurately, but their high cost may make them insufficiently cost-effective for general use.

A risk-factor profile is a useful indicator – the more risk factors that apply to you from the above list, the greater the risk of osteoporosis.

Effects of HRT on osteoporosis

Oestrogens
Oestrogen therapy prevents or reduces bone loss, if it is taken soon after the menopause, before osteoporosis has become established. If you take HRT for at least five years, the risk is reduced by up to 50 per cent. Studies show that the number of cases of hip fractures in women aged 60–69 using HRT for five years is 4–5 per 1,000 women versus 7–8 per 1,000 women not using HRT. For women aged 60–69 who have used HRT for ten years, the risk is reduced to 2–3 per 1,000 women. So the longer you take HRT, the better protection you get – if you are at high risk of osteoporosis, it may be necessary to take it lifelong.

Progestogens
Several studies suggest that progestogens taken alone, without oestrogen, can prevent bone loss. Other studies refute this finding, so more research is needed to ascertain exactly what the long-term benefits and side-effects are, before its use can be recommended.

Established osteoporosis

Oestrogen, with or without progesterone, appears to be effective even in patients with established osteoporosis. Some studies found that bone mass increased by as much as 6.4 per cent each year, though this may not be of good-quality bone and so would have little effect on reducing the risk of fractures.

Colorectal cancer

Recent research has shown that the risk of colorectal cancer in women using HRT for five years between the ages of 60 and 69 is 5 per 1,000 women versus a risk of 8 per 1,000 non-users. After ten years HRT, the risk is further reduced to 2–3 per 1,000 women.

Dementia

Recent studies suggest that replacing oestrogens after the menopause may have a direct effect on general blood flow in the brain. In the long term, oestrogen replacement may help to prevent dementia and Alzheimer's disease. Furthermore, oestrogens may improve cognition in women who already have the disease.

Other benefits

There is some evidence that HRT use may be associated with reduced tooth loss, reduced incidence of age-related macular degeneration and cataracts of the eyes, improved bowel continence, improved wound healing and improved balance. However, more research is necessary to confirm these findings.

Women at most risk of oestrogen deficiency

Early menopause

The average age at the menopause is 51. If you experience the menopause before the age of 40, it is defined as an early menopause. About 1 per cent of women have an early menopause, that is about 100,000 women in the UK alone.

The age at menopause tends to follow a pattern through the female line. If your mother had an early menopause, the same is likely for you, and your daughter.

In most cases of an early menopause, the ovaries stop functioning without any identifiable cause. Occasionally there is evidence of auto immune disease, where the body sees the ovaries as 'foreign' and tries to destroy them. In some cases, this can affect the ovaries. Occasionally auto immune ovarian failure is linked to other auto immune conditions, most commonly thyroid disease. In a small number of women, the ovaries never developed properly in the first place, or the intricate hormonal cycle between the hypothalamus, pituitary and ovaries has been upset, often by severe illness. Surgery, chemotherapy or radiotherapy can also affect the normal working of the ovaries.

Whatever the reason, an early menopause causes infertility as well as all the symptoms and long-term consequences of oestrogen deficiency. Of prime importance is the increased risk of osteoporosis. Oestrogen replacement therapy can treat the symptoms of the menopause and help prevent osteoporosis. Most doctors recommend that if you have had an early menopause, you should take oestrogen therapy at least until your fifty-first birthday – the usual age at menopause – and possibly lifelong.

Hysterectomy

Removal of the uterus (hysterectomy) is increasingly recommended for older women to treat heavy and irregular periods, fibroids or cancer. In most cases only the uterus is removed, and the ovaries are left. This is to ensure the continued production of oestrogen from the ovaries, until the time of the natural menopause.

If you are nearing the age of 50 when you have a hysterectomy, or are post-menopausal, the doctor may remove your ovaries as well, even if they are healthy. Removal of the ovaries would then prevent any future risk (however small) of ovarian cancer.

Before the 1970s it was fairly common for the ovaries to be removed at hysterectomy, whatever the age of the woman. Women who have had a 'total hysterectomy' as it is called, will experience a 'surgical menopause' with all the symptoms of oestrogen withdrawal, immediately following the operation. Unfortunately, in those days HRT was not routinely prescribed; at that time little was known about the greater risks of heart disease and osteoporosis if the menopause occurred before a woman reached the age of 40.

Even if your ovaries remain, it is not the end of the problem. After the operation, the ovaries continue to function normally, even though you will no longer have periods. Eventually they stop working, just as at the natural menopause. Research shows that, on average, removing the uterus causes the ovaries to stop functioning about four years earlier than the normal menopause. In one study, 25 per cent of women suffered ovarian failure within two years of hysterectomy.

It follows that if you have had a hysterectomy, with or without removal of your ovaries, you should carefully consider your risk of osteoporosis. Because cancer of the uterus is no longer a threat, you can take oestrogen on its own, without the need for progestogens. As with an early natural menopause, doctors suggest you take oestrogen at least until the age of 51, and possibly for longer.

Summary

- Hormone replacement therapy effectively treats many of the symptoms of the menopause.
- If you take HRT, it will reduce the likelihood of osteoporosis, but you need to consider lifelong treatment.
- HRT has been shown to prevent the risk of dementia and Alzheimer's disease, and may also help to treat these conditions.
- HRT reduces the risk of colorectal cancer.
- It is important to consider taking HRT if you have an early menopause, especially before the age of 40, or if you have a hysterectomy. Both of these factors increase your risk of osteoporosis.

6

Potential Problems – Risk versus Benefit

There are two main reasons why women decide against HRT and, indeed, why some doctors choose not to prescribe it. The first reason is the side-effects: for example, nausea, breast tenderness, and especially the nuisance of monthly 'periods' necessary in some regimens. The other reason is the fear that HRT causes cancer.

Every effective drug has some unwanted effects. The objective of modern therapy is to enhance the benefits of HRT and reduce the risks.

Hormone replacement does not exactly re-create the pre-menopausal state. It is impossible to mimic the complex hormonal changes that make up the normal menstrual cycle. For a start, oestrogen levels fluctuate during the menstrual cycle, with a peak just before ovulation. Some regimes of HRT try to copy these fluctuations, but most do not. Furthermore, the different types of hormones used in HRT and the different regimens all have varying effects.

This first section of the chapter discusses the possible side-effects of HRT and ways of minimizing them if they have not improved after the first few months of treatment.

The second part deals with the reasons why some women should not take HRT, and the potential risks of taking HRT. Several 'relative' risks are discussed – certain medical conditions that can be aggravated by HRT, for example gallstones.

The major fear about HRT is the risk of cancer, and this is addressed in the final section of the chapter.

The settling down period

It can take up to three months of therapy before benefits are noticed, and side-effects frequently appear before the positive effects. Fortunately many of the side-effects, particularly bloating, breast tenderness and nausea, usually settle down after the first few months of treatment so it is important not to stop HRT until you have given it a fair trial.

Side-effects of hormone replacement therapy

All drugs have side-effects and hormone replacement therapy is no exception. Some of these are the result of oestrogen, others are due to progestogen. Not every woman taking HRT will necessarily experience all, or even any, of these effects.

Withdrawal bleeding: the return of 'periods'
Bleeding is a problem of most regimes for perimenopausal women who have a uterus. It occurs with regimens of oestrogens alone, and oestrogen combined with progestogen. About 85 per cent of women will have a 'period' – the withdrawal bleed – if they take a course of progestogen for twelve days each month. This bleed usually starts near the end of the oral progestogen course and lasts between four and seven days. This may be acceptable to most 50-year-old women but is often intolerable ten years later, particularly by women starting HRT for the first time. The good news is that after the natural menopause women can switch to a continuous combined 'period-free' regimen. This still gives protection from the risk of cancer of the uterus – it is just that the lining of the uterus has not been stimulated enough to thicken, and there is nothing to shed.

Continuous combined HRT is not generally recommended before the menopause as a woman's own hormones can override the HRT resulting in irregular or heavy bleeding, particularly in the early stages. Obviously it can be difficult to tell when the natural menopause occurs in women taking HRT but since most women have stopped their natural periods by around 54, women using cyclical HRT can often be switched to 'period-free' HRT at this time.

Irregular bleeding
Irregular bleeding, or breakthrough bleeding, is any unexpected bleeding from the vagina. It is common in the first months of treatment, usually establishing a regular pattern by the third month.

It is rarely due to anything sinister, the commonest reasons being:

- Missing a dose – forgetting to take the tablets one or two days in a row, or not changing the patch at the right time is the commonest cause of breakthrough bleeding.
- Diarrhoea or vomiting – this prevents the absorption of oestrogen and progestogen into the body so the effects are the same as

forgetting to take the tablets. This is only a problem for oral treatment.

- Antibiotics – these may reduce the effect of HRT, resulting in breakthrough bleeding.
- Treatment for epilepsy – some of the drugs used to control epilepsy, e.g. phenytoin, cause the oestrogen to be cleared from the body much more quickly than usual, reducing the effects of HRT.
- Stress – in the same way as stress can provoke an irregular menstrual cycle during the reproductive years, it can also upset the balance of HRT.
- Long-distance travel – especially if it includes a change in time zones as the delicate balance of the body's own hormonal clock is disrupted.

Leg cramps

These affect both legs and tend to be worse at night. They are most noticeable during the first few weeks after starting HRT. The reasons for the cramps remain a mystery but studies show that they are not due to thromboses. However, you should see your doctor if the pain only affects one leg.

Painful or tender breasts

Breasts become swollen and tender because of the hormonal stimulation from both oestrogen and progestogen. This usually improves after a few months of treatment.

Weight changes

Most women do not gain weight when taking HRT, and some women even lose it. In most cases, any weight gain is due to water retention, not an increase in body fat, and usually settles down after the first few months of treatment. However, a few women do experience a sudden weight increase that disappears when oestrogens are discontinued.

Nausea

Nausea appears to be more of a problem for women taking oral oestrogens. Sometimes taking the tablets with food or at bedtime gives relief. If not, it is worth trying a different route of treatment.

Vaginal discharge
Oestrogen stimulates the glands of the cervix, producing a lubricating vaginal discharge.

Eye irritation
A few women find that their contact lenses become uncomfortable. This effect of oestrogen also happens during pregnancy, and to women taking the oral contraceptive pill.

Skin irritation
High doses of oestrogen can occasionally make the skin feel itchy. A few women find that the oestrogen patches irritate their skin.

The pre-menstrual syndrome
Cyclical progestogens frequently cause symptoms similar to the premenstrual syndrome:

- breast tenderness;
- nausea;
- depression;
- irritability;
- stomach cramps;
- water retention.

Up to 20 to 30 per cent of women notice these symptoms; especially those who suffered from the pre-menstrual syndrome, and they often peak towards the end of the progestogen phases, just before the 'period'. Most women experiencing these problems with one type of progestogen benefit from changing to another type or route. Only about 5 per cent of women are sensitive to all types of progestogens. Natural progesterone, either as a pessary/suppository or vaginal gel, is a possible alternative.

Headaches
Headaches are a common problem for women during the menopause, and many women start to notice a link between their migraine attacks and periods during the years building up to the menopause. There are very few studies of the effects of HRT on headaches and migraine, and different regimens probably have different effects. It might be worthwhile trying a different type of HRT if headaches become a problem.

There is no reason why women with migraine should not take HRT but it should be stopped, or perhaps an alternative type of HRT tried, if the attacks become more frequent or severe. If migraine aura develops after starting HRT, discuss with your doctor about reducing the dose of oestrogen or, if you are taking tablets, changing to a non-oral method.

Lack of effect

Occasionally HRT fails to control the menopausal symptoms. Increasing the dose is usually sufficient to solve the problems. A few women taking oral treatment do not absorb the hormones and need to change to patches or implants.

Fibroids

Thickening of the lining of the womb, the endometrium, is prevented by progestogens. Long-term oestrogen stimulation in the absence of progestogens can cause fibroids to enlarge, which may cause heavy bleeding.

HRT – a drug of addiction?

Dr Thomas Bewley, a former President of the Royal College of Psychiatrists, and his daughter Dr Susan Bewley, a gynaecologist, published an article in *The Lancet* expressing their concern that some women might become dependent on HRT. They argued that oestrogens can lift mood and have other powerful psychological effects. The media picked up on this, with the inaccurate headline 'HRT can be as addictive as heroin' appearing on the front page of *The Times*. The Drs Bewley were only alerting people to the possibility of dependence, not inferring that every woman is addicted to HRT.

It is possible, particularly with implants, to become accustomed to artificially high levels of oestrogen. As the implant wears off, symptoms return at increasingly shorter intervals. These symptoms are due to the falling levels of oestrogen; adjusting the treatment can sort these problems out and prevent this happening again.

What can you do if you suffer severe side-effects?

Obviously the first thing to do is speak to your doctor. There are five possible strategies:

- reduce the dose of oestrogen or progestogen;
- change to a different type or route of progestogen;
- consider natural progesterone;

- reduce the duration of progestogen therapy each month;
- hysterectomy.

Side-effects can be related to the dose you take; starting treatment with the lowest dose will minimize any problems. Similarly, the type of progestogen can be changed; sometimes it may be necessary to try two or three different ones. You can also change the regimen of taking HRT – for example, if you are taking a combined oestrogen/progestogen course of ten or twelve days of progestogens every month (cyclical regime), you may find switching to oestrogen and progestogen tablets taken every day (continuous combined regime) causes fewer problems. It is possible to take progestogen for fewer days each month but this does reduce the protection against cancer of the uterus and so is not recommended. The levonorgestrel intrauterine system (Mirena®) is an alternative method of protecting the lining of the womb in women who cannot tolerate other forms of progestogen and also
provides effective contraception by releasing very low doses of progestogen directly into the womb. This means that very little progestogen gets into the circulation. At the time of writing its licensed indication is for contraception and heavy periods although it is widely used for HRT. Progesterone vaginal gel can be useful for women who experience side-effects with synthetic progestogens. Progesterone is also available as pessaries or suppositories. However, they need to be used twice daily and sedation is a common problem.

The risks of HRT

The major risk of HRT is that of cancer, especially breast cancer and cancer of the uterus. There is always the risk of these cancers, whether or not you take HRT. Research aims to find out if HRT increases the risk.

The problem with research

The benefits of HRT are already reflected in the lower death rates among users compared to non-users. However, some of the information on the protective effects of HRT – and the possible risks – comes from studies noting the incidence of these conditions in women taking HRT: that is, the number of women who experience any of the conditions under study while taking treatment. This is then compared to the expected incidence if they had not taken HRT.

Such studies have obvious inherent limitations and do not always reflect accurately the effects of HRT. It is difficult to assess the risks and benefits of HRT alone, as the diseases it helps to prevent are affected by numerous different factors. For example, heart disease is affected by genetic make up, general health, diet and exercise. It is almost impossible to single out the effect of HRT as, besides its direct action on preventing heart disease, women taking HRT often change their diet and make greater efforts to improve their general health.

Moreover, lifestyle and diet might be intrinsically different in women choosing to take HRT, before they even start treatment. In some studies, women taking HRT tended to be from higher social classes than non-users. This could make HRT seem more effective than it really is as these women tend to be healthier and have a lower risk of heart disease, even before they take oestrogen.

At the simplest level, studies need to compare the effects of HRT, taken for several years, with a control group of women, of the same age and social background, who have not taken HRT.

Risk versus benefit

For women at high risk of osteoporosis, HRT may be a life-saver. But HRT does not suit all women, nor should it be recommended for every woman. Long-term use of HRT may increase the risk of some potentially serious conditions such as breast and other cancers. Although for a long time HRT was considered to protect against heart disease and stroke, recent evidence refutes these claims for certain types of HRT, which may in fact increase the risk of these conditions. It is important to remember that all these conditions can occur whether or not you use HRT, and the decision to take HRT really depends on your own set of personal risks and potential benefits.

Coronary heart disease and strokes

It is quite rare for a woman to suffer a heart attack or a stroke before the menopause; the incidence starts to rise in post-menopausal women. Heart disease is now recognized as the leading cause of early death in women, more significant than any single type of cancer. Twenty per cent of women are at risk of stroke, with an 8 per cent chance of death. Likewise, women have a 46 per cent chance of developing coronary heart disease and a one in three chance of death.

A large study in the USA has followed the health of more than 120,000 nurses since 1976. By 1986, almost 50,000 of them had passed through the menopause and about one half of them had taken HRT. In those taking HRT, the rate of death from heart disease was 39 per cent less than the non-takers. The amount of coronary artery disease diagnosed among users was only 51 per cent that of non-users. These figures, showing the benefit for women taking HRT, strongly suggest that the menopause itself is a severe risk factor for heart disease.

Who is at risk of heart disease and stroke?

Lists of risk factors are traditionally used as means of estimating the chances of developing heart disease. Various different factors are assessed, including lifestyle and medical history. In general, the greater the number of factors present, the higher the risk. These charts are useful for assessing the overall risk in a specific group of people. They are of little predictive value when applied to individuals, but can highlight those most at risk.

Risk factors for heart disease and stroke include:

- age;
- sex;
- a blood relative with heart disease;
- high blood pressure;
- smoking;
- high cholesterol;
- diabetes;
- angina;
- obesity;
- lack of exercise.

Age

The risk of heart disease progressively increases with age.

Sex

Men are at much greater risk than pre-menopausal women. After the menopause, the risk for women increases.

Family history

Heart disease frequently affects several members of the same family. This could be because of a genetic link, or because they share a similar diet and lifestyle.

High blood pressure
Hypertension is associated with a high risk of heart disease. Treatment with drugs to lower the blood pressure reduces the risk of strokes but seems to have little effect on heart attacks.

Smoking
In men, the effect of smoking is directly related to the number of cigarettes smoked. This relationship is not so obvious in women, but smoking is still an important factor.

High cholesterol
High cholesterol levels are strongly linked to an increased risk of heart disease. Lowering the cholesterol can reduce the risk.

Diabetes
Diabetes is associated with generalized disease of the blood vessels, which increases the risk of heart disease.

Angina
Angina is a gripping pain in the centre of the chest, often provoked by exercise and relieved by rest. Since the pain is evidence of restricted blood flow to the heart muscle, angina indicates a high risk of having a heart attack.

Obesity
Obesity is a difficult risk factor to assess as it is linked with other risk factors: women who take little exercise or who have high blood pressure are often also overweight. Several members of the same family groups are frequently overweight, and may be affected by heart disease.

Exercise
Lack of exercise increases the risk of heart disease; regular exercise reduces the risk. Starting an exercise programme is often linked with a change to a healthier diet, both of which can reduce cholesterol levels and blood pressure.

You cannot do much about certain risk factors for heart disease, such as age and family history – for example, if you have a relative who died young from heart disease. Yet if you are at risk, you can do something about the other major factors such as raised cholesterol levels, obesity, high blood pressure and smoking.

Screening for risk factors of heart disease

Obesity

Obesity can be assessed using tables of ideal weight for any given height. More than 10 per cent over the ideal weight is classified as overweight, 20 per cent or more is classified as obesity.

A more accurate measurement is based on your Body Mass Index (BMI), also called the Quatelet index. This can easily be calculated using the following formula:

Body Mass Index = weight (kg)/(height in metres)^2

This gives a simple numerical index. A woman's ideal BMI should be between 19 and 25. You are underweight if the index is less than 19, and overweight if it is more than 25.

Cholesterol

Another screening test for heart disease is to measure the level of cholesterol in your blood. This should be done not less than twelve hours after the last meal. The average level of cholesterol is between 3.5 and 6.5 mmol per litre of blood plasma. Ideally, the level should be under 5.2 mmol per litre.

The cholesterol story

As you get older, fatty deposits called atheroma build up in the walls of the blood vessels. In time this fat starts to harden. Eventually the fat narrows the vessel, blocking the normal flow of blood. If the blood vessels supplying the heart are involved, the result is coronary heart disease, giving rise to angina or a heart attack. Strokes can result if the blood vessels supplying the brain are affected.

Cholesterol is a special type of fat. High levels of cholesterol are linked to heart disease. It is carried in the bloodstream, bound to special proteins called *low density lipoproteins* (LDL). These proteins deposit the cholesterol in the walls of arteries, where it accumulates and hardens, causing atheroma. Other carrier proteins, called *high density lipoproteins* (HDL), protect against heart disease by transporting the cholesterol away from the walls of the artery, back to the liver.

59

Effects of HRT on heart disease

Oestrogen has a protective effect by causing both the level of cholesterol in the bloodstream, and the level of the low density lipoproteins associated with atheroma, to fall. It also increases the amount of protective high density lipoproteins.

Unfortunately, real life is much more complex than this. Although a number of studies have confirmed that oestrogen replacement does reduce the risk of heart disease, possibly by as much as 50 per cent, it is now thought that some of this benefit may have been due to selection bias – healthier women took HRT. Recent studies have shown that some types of HRT, those that contain conjugated oestrogens and medroxyprogesterone acetate, do not prevent heart disease and may increase the risk for heart disease in the first year of taking them.

The bottom line is that the true effect of other types of HRT remains unknown. More studies are needed; different oestrogens and progestogens – both type and route of administration – are likely to have different effects on the risk.

See your doctor **immediately** *if*:

- you experience unexplained episodes of chest pain, with or without sweating, breathlessness or dizziness.

Effects of HRT on stroke

A stroke occurs when the blood supply to the brain is blocked (thrombotic stroke) or when blood leaks from a blood vessel in the brain (haemorrhagic stroke). Strokes can be caused by a build-up of atherosclerosis in blood vessels, similar to heart disease. Therefore, the same risk factors of high blood pressure, smoking, excessive alcohol, etc., also apply to stroke. It was thought that HRT had little effect on stroke but recent research suggests that HRT may slightly increase the likelihood of stroke. About 3 out of 1,000 women in their fifties not using HRT can expect to have a stroke in any five-year period. For women of a similar age who use HRT for five years, the figure rises to 4 per 1,000. Age is itself a risk factor for stroke so the risk in non-HRT users in their sixties is 11 per 1,000 in any five-year period versus 15 per 1,000 women of the same age using HRT.

See your doctor **immediately** *if*:

- you experience any unusual migraine-type symptoms or unusual faints or limb weakness.

Venous thrombosis (VTE or DVT)

Blood clots can sometimes form in the veins, typically in the calf, causing a swollen, red limb. In most cases clots are successfully treated with anticoagulants. Rarely, a clot can move into the lungs, known as a pulmonary embolism (PE), resulting in breathlessness, chest pains and collapse, with fatal consequences.

Risk factors for venous thrombosis

- A close relative with venous thrombosis under age 45.
- Obesity.
- Immobility (e.g. surgery or wheelchair-bound).
- Severe varicose veins.

Effects of HRT

Increasing age is the main risk for venous thrombosis although research suggests that women using HRT are more likely to develop venous thrombosis than women of a similar age who are not using HRT, especially in the first year of use. About 3 per 1,000 women in their fifties who do not use HRT are likely to have a venous thrombosis in any five-year period compared to 7 per 1,000 women of the same age who take HRT. By the time they reach their sixties the risk in non-users increases to 8 per 1,000 women in a five-year period compared to 17 per 1,000 women taking HRT.

If you, or a close relative, have had an unexplained venous thrombosis at a young age, you may need to have a blood test to check your blood clotting before you can take HRT. If you have major surgery and will be off your feet for a while, you may be advised to stop HRT 4–6 weeks before your operation to reduce your risks of venous thrombosis. You can start the HRT again once you are fully mobile.

See your doctor if:

- you experience a red, swollen, tender calf for no apparent reason;
- you experience sharp chest pains or breathlessness.

Breast cancer

There is a one in ten chance that a woman will have breast cancer during her lifetime. It used to be the commonest type of cancer in women but lung cancer now holds top position. Both oestrogens and progesterone produced by the ovaries affect breast cancer, but there are numerous other factors associated with its development. As a general rule, the larger the number of risk factors that apply to you, the greater the risk of developing breast cancer. This is by no means a hard and fast rule – it should only be used as an indicator.

Risk factors for breast cancer
- An early menarche.
- A late menopause.
- Obesity.
- A close relative with breast cancer.
- Having no children.
- Late age at first full-term pregnancy.

Possible risk factors
- A high fat diet.
- Alcohol.
- Benign breast disease – non-cancerous breast lumps.

Protective factors
- Removal of the ovaries before the menopause.
- Young age at first full-term pregnancy.

Effects of HRT
Most doctors believe that taking HRT for up to five years does not seem to increase the risk of breast cancer. After five years, the risk increases the longer you take it. Any excess risk should be balanced against the background risk of breast cancer in non-users; an estimated 45 per 1,000 women not using HRT develop breast cancer by the age of 70. For women taking HRT for five years, the risk increases by 2 per 1,000 women. For women taking HRT for ten years, the risk increases by 6 per 1,000 women.

It is not all bad news: the risk returns to the background risk by five years after stopping HRT. Furthermore, the risk of death from breast cancer is no different from non-users, and may even be less; the cancer in HRT users seems less likely to spread to other parts of the body. Regular breast checks also lead to earlier detection in HRT users, increasing chances of survival.

See your doctor if:

- you notice any changes to your breast such as lumps, skin changes or nipple discharge.

Cancer of the womb lining (endometrium)

From a group of 1,000 post-menopausal women who were not on HRT, only one would be expected to get cancer of the womb. With the modern regime of HRT which combines oestrogen replacement with progestogen, the risk of uterine cancer is at least the same as this, if not lower.

Risk factors for cancer of the womb

There are several groups of women for whom the risk is increased. They involve:

- obesity;
- women who do not ovulate regularly;
- oestrogen replacement 'unopposed' by progestogens in women who have not had a hysterectomy.

Obesity

Fat women continue to produce more oestrogen after the menopause than thinner women, since the male hormones that the ovaries produce after the menopause are converted to oestrogen in the fat cells. Because of this, fatter women are less at risk of osteoporosis, but have a greater risk of uterine cancer – the higher levels of oestrogens stimulate the lining of the uterus.

Failure to ovulate regularly

One reason for irregular menstrual cycles is a failure to ovulate regularly. Such 'anovulatory' cycles are not uncommon during the climacteric. This can increase the risk of uterine cancer: if an egg is not released from the ovary, the progesterone levels do not rise in the second part of the menstrual cycle and the lining of the uterus is over-stimulated by the oestrogen.

'Unopposed' oestrogens

In the same way, oestrogen therapy, 'unopposed' by progestogens, leads to abnormal thickening of the lining of the uterus – endometrial hyperplasia – and cancer. If progestogens are not taken, 7 per cent of women taking low doses of oestrogen develop endometrial hyperplasia, rising to 15 per cent at higher doses. Endometrial hyperplasia is a cause of irregular heavy bleeding and carries a small but significant risk (1 per cent) of turning cancerous.

This cancer is usually of a particular type, called adenocarcinoma, which responds well to treatment: if you develop this type of cancer and are treated, you have a 99 per cent chance of survival. Another type of cancer, atypical hyperplasia, is much more rare and does not respond so well to treatment.

Unopposed oestrogen treatment has a prolonged carry-over effect and the increased risk remains for many years after it has been discontinued. Even fifteen years after stopping treatment, the risk of cancer of the uterus is still six times greater than the average risk.

Fortunately, the effect of unopposed oestrogens can be prevented and usually reversed by treatment with cyclical progestogen – one study showed that the progestogen norethisterone, taken for 21 days a month for three months, converted the endometrium of all women with endometrial hyperplasia back to normal.

This protective effect means that many doctors refuse to prescribe unopposed oestrogens to women with a uterus. The amount of protection depends on the number of days that the progestogens are taken for every 28 days of oestrogen therapy: 3 per cent of women get endometrial hyperplasia if they take seven days of progestogen therapy each month, 2 per cent with ten days, and none with 12 to 13 days of progestogen.

Because of this, it is recommended that progestogens are taken for at least 12 days out of every 28. This usually leads to a 'period' near the end of the course. Even if there is no bleeding, you are still protected.

Paradoxically, women who do develop endometrial cancer while taking oestrogen still have a lower overall death rate than women of a similar age who do not have cancer. This is probably due, at least in part, to a lower risk of heart disease among women who take oestrogen.

See your doctor if:

* you notice any new vaginal bleeding several months after starting HRT. Although it is common to experience bleeding and spotting within the first few months of starting HRT, this usually settles with continued use. Therefore any new or unusual bleeding starting after this time should be reported to your doctor.

Cancer of the ovaries

There appears to be a small increase in risk of ovarian cancer in women using oestrogen-only HRT for more than five years. The background risk in non-users aged 50–69 is 9 per 1,000 women, which rises to 10 per 1,000 women after five years' use of HRT and to 12 per 1,000 women after ten years' HRT. The effect of long-term combined oestrogen–progestogen HRT on ovarian cancer is not known.

See your doctor if:

- you experience any abdominal swelling and discomfort, weight loss and/or abnormal vaginal bleeding, possibly associated with an abdominal lump. These symptoms do not necessarily mean that you have an ovarian cancer – more commonly they are due to non-cancerous ovarian cysts which will respond to treatment.

Cancer of the cervix

There is no evidence that cancer of the cervix is affected by HRT. In fact, women with cancer of the cervix are a frequently neglected group who would benefit from HRT because it keeps the tissues moist, making it easier for doctors to interpret cervical smear tests.

HRT and pre-existing medical problems

There are very few reasons why a woman might not be able to start HRT. Such reasons include:
- hormone-related cancers: cancer of the womb (endometrium), breast cancer;
- active liver disease;
- blood clots, i.e. venous thrombosis or pulmonary embolism;
- strokes or heart disease;
- irregular vaginal bleeding of unknown cause;
- pregnancy.

Women who have, or have had, womb cancer

One of the treatments for cancer of the womb is to remove the ovaries. This is because many doctors think that the high levels of oestrogens produced by the ovaries stimulate the cancer to grow. Unfortunately, removing the ovaries can cause severe menopausal symptoms. Even women who have their ovaries removed several years after the menopause experience symptoms. This is probably because after the menopause the ovaries continue to produce the male hormones, androgens, which are converted to oestrogen. If the woman is producing high levels of androgens, removing the ovaries will cause oestrogen levels to fall, producing menopausal symptoms.

One type of cancer of the womb can develop from the condition endometrial hyperplasia, when the lining of the uterus – the endometrium – has been over-stimulated by oestrogen, without the opposing effects of progesterone. Some doctors have found that if this cancer is treated at a very early stage, women who receive HRT after treatment live longer than women who do not.

In light of this discovery the American College of Obstetricians and Gynaecologists has issued a Committee Opinion, suggesting that women who have been treated for cancer of the womb should be offered HRT for the same reasons as any other women. Nevertheless, they stress the importance of individualization of treatment, assessing the risks versus the benefits for each woman. Until further studies confirm these findings, HRT is best avoided by women who have had cancer of the uterus, unless they seek expert advice.

Women who currently have endometrial hyperplasia, or who have already developed cancer, should not take oestrogen as it can stimulate the cancer to grow. However, many doctors recommend a hysterectomy, after which it is safe to take HRT. Progestogens are sometimes prescribed in addition to oestrogen, despite hysterectomy.

Women who have, or have had, breast cancer

Circumstantial evidence suggests that there are few reasons why a woman successfully treated for breast cancer cannot take HRT. In the past there was concern that high levels of oestrogen stimulated growth of the cancer. Because of this, many women had their ovaries removed as part of the treatment for breast cancer, in order to reduce the natural levels of oestrogen. However, studies show that there is little difference in the long-term survival rates between women who have had their ovaries removed and those who have not.

Furthermore, women with a history of breast cancer were often advised against becoming pregnant, because of concern about high oestrogen levels during pregnancy. Again, recent data does not back this up.

HRT may even have specific advantages: some women treated for breast cancer have substantially higher overall risks from the effects of osteoporosis than from the recurrence of breast cancer.

HRT and the treatment of breast cancer

The standard treatment of breast cancer is with anti-oestrogen drugs, such as tamoxifen. It can hasten the onset of the menopause, causing such severe menopausal symptoms that many women stop taking it. Trials are underway giving HRT to women taking anti-oestrogens, in the hope of preventing the hot flushes, night sweats and other menopausal problems. Evidence suggests that drugs such as tamoxifen can still halt the growth of the tumour, even in the presence of oestrogen.

But the woman's own choice is always an important factor, even when there may be clear risks involved in treatment. Therefore, although HRT is not generally advised for women who have, or have had, breast cancer, its use may be justified in certain cases, guided by a specialist menopause clinic or oncologist.

Active liver disease

HRT should not be taken by women with jaundice due to severe liver disease as most of the oestrogen, particularly if taken by mouth, is broken down by the liver. If the jaundice improves and liver works normally again, there is no reason why HRT should not be taken then. Some doctors feel it is safer to use the non-oral form – patches or implants – as most of the oral dose is processed by the liver.

Women who have, or have had, venous thrombosis or pulmonary embolism

A personal history of venous thrombosis is the single biggest risk factor for a further event, with or without HRT. Because unexplained venous thrombosis can result from a clotting disorder, or thrombophilia, investigations to screen for a thrombophilia or underlying disease may be necessary before HRT can be considered. Even if this is negative, HRT should still be used with caution.

Women who have, or have had, strokes or heart disease

In light of recent evidence, HRT is not generally recommended for the prevention of heart disease and strokes, although it may be given to women with a past history of such an event if they have severe menopausal symptoms or are at risk of osteoporosis.

Irregular or heavy periods

Women who have irregular or heavy periods need to be carefully checked to rule out any underlying cause of the bleeding before starting HRT.

Pregnancy

The menopause is a dangerous time as many women with irregular periods frequently assume that they no longer need to use contraceptives; if a woman's periods stop, she may assume it is the menopause, and not realize that she is pregnant. Doctors recommend that contraception is continued for at least twelve months after the last period in women over the age of 50. Women who have an earlier menopause are advised to continue contraception for at least two years. It is unlikely that HRT would have much effect if it had been taken in early pregnancy, although there are no studies to confirm this.

Other medical conditions that can be affected by HRT

HRT can also aggravate other medical conditions such as gall bladder disease, endometriosis, fibroids and non-cancerous breast disease. In all these cases, the decision to take HRT depends on individual circumstances. You need to discuss the severity of your symptoms with your doctor, and balance the long-term benefits of HRT against the risks of treatment.

Gallstones

HRT should be used cautiously by women with gallstones as they may enlarge, particularly with oral therapy. If you have had problems with gallstones in the past, some doctors suggest you should use patches or implants rather than tablets. It is safe to use HRT if you have had an operation to remove gallstones.

Endometriosis

Sometimes the tissue that lines the uterus is found in abnormal sites. In the same way that the lining of the uterus is shed each month during menstruation, these other sites also bleed, causing severe pain and heavy periods. This condition, known as endometriosis, is stimulated by oestrogen and improves with the menopause. HRT can occasionally reactivate the condition so women who have had endometriosis should be cautious when taking HRT, monitoring any symptoms particularly of pain on intercourse and heavy or irregular bleeding.

Fibroids

Fibroids – non-cancerous growths in the muscle of the uterus – are very common. They are sensitive to oestrogen so often grow during pregnancy as the level of oestrogen in the body rises, and shrink after the menopause. Because of this, fibroids can enlarge with HRT, causing heavy withdrawal bleeding.

High blood pressure

Women being treated for high blood pressure can take HRT; natural oestrogens do not affect blood pressure in the majority of women with high or normal blood pressure, and may even lower it. However, about 5 per cent of post-menopausal women have a rare sensitivity, particularly to the equine oestrogens, and their blood pressure goes up. This does not rule out trying non-oral forms of oestrogen.

Diabetes

If the diabetes is well controlled, there is no reason why you should not take HRT, but you should monitor your blood sugar carefully when you start treatment, and make a note of any unusual symptoms. Non-oral routes are generally recommended.

Otosclerosis

Otosclerosis is an inherited cause of hearing loss caused by the growth of extra bone that prevents the small bones in the ear from working properly. This condition can deteriorate rapidly during pregnancy, suggesting a link with oestrogen. HRT may have the same effect, so specialist advice should be sought before starting treatment.

Varicose veins

If these are extensive, it might be advisable not to take HRT. Treatment should be stopped if they become painful or inflamed.

Migraine

The effect of HRT on migraine is unpredictable – some women notice a great improvement, others have more frequent attacks. The attacks often seem to link to oestrogen fluctuations, particularly if tablets are missed or taken at a different time from usual. Sometimes attacks link to the progestogen phase of the HRT. The migraine may settle down after the first few months of treatment as the body adapts to the hormones, so persevere with HRT for a few months before discontinuing. Changing to a different type or route of oestrogen, particularly patches or the gel, may be worth trying. If attacks link to the progestogen phase, changing to a different progestogen may help. Some women develop migraine aura soon after starting HRT. In these cases the dose of HRT should be reduced or you should change to a non-oral route.

Thyroid disease
Women with an overactive thyroid are at increased risk of osteoporosis and hip fracture. HRT can be of great benefit to reduce this risk, although the dose of thyroxine may need to be increased when HRT is started.

Breast lumps
If you have breast lumps, they should be checked by your doctor to make sure they are not cancerous, before starting HRT. Regular checks should be continued once treatment has begun.

Summary

- The usual reasons for stopping treatment are side-effects – particularly bleeding and effects of progestogen therapy.
- Many of the initial side-effects settle after a few months of treatment.
- If side-effects do not settle, it is worthwhile altering the dose of hormones, trying an alternative route, changing the progestogen, or following a different regime.
- There are very few reasons why any woman cannot take HRT.
- There is a slight increased risk of breast cancer and perhaps ovarian cancer and stroke from long-term use of HRT.
- Certain types of HRT containing conjugated oestrogens and medroxyprogesterone acetate do not prevent heart disease and may increase the chances of a heart attack in the first year of use.
- HRT may increase the risk of venous thrombosis, particularly in the first year of use.

7

Pills, Patches, Gels, Nasal Spray, Vaginal Rings or Implants?

HRT is a combination of the two female hormones: oestrogen and progesterone. The oestrogen effectively treats the symptoms of the menopause; progesterone is necessary to prevent the oestrogen over-stimulating the lining of the uterus – the endometrium – which can lead to cancer. Unless you have had a hysterectomy, it is important to take both hormones. They may be administered by several different routes: tablets taken daily, patches changed every couple of days, a daily nasal spray, vaginal rings, or implants inserted under the skin and replaced at six-month intervals.

Oestrogens used in modern hormonal therapy are either *natural* or *synthetic*.

- *Natural* oestrogens include *oestradiol*, *oestrone* and *oestriol*. These are the same oestrogens that the ovaries produce. Most of these oestrogens are artificially manufactured for use as HRT; they are still termed 'natural' because they have exactly the same effects as the oestrogens normally found in the body.
- *Synthetic* oestrogens include *ethinyloestradiol*, *mestranol* and *stilboestrol*. They have a different chemical structure to the natural oestrogens but are more potent. Synthetic oestrogens are used for contraception, as they prevent ovulation – the monthly release of an egg from one of the ovaries. Unfortunately, synthetic oestrogens can affect the production of blood-clotting factors more than natural oestrogens, increasing the risk of thrombosis. In general, only natural oestrogens are used to treat the menopause.

Natural progesterone is rapidly broken down in the body and has to be taken several times a day to be effective. For this reason, synthetic progesterone – progestogen – is usually used both for contraception and for HRT as only a single daily dose is necessary. There are several different types of progestogens, which have differing advantages and disadvantages.

The choice between different types of HRT is enormous: as well as the many different oestrogens and progestogens, there are different routes – pills, patches, gels, nasal spray, vaginal rings and implants – and different regimens – cyclical or continuous.

Oestrogens

Of the three oestrogens produced by the ovaries, *oestradiol* is the most potent, and *oestriol* the least. The early forms of HRT used oral natural oestrogens which the body rapidly inactivates: they are absorbed from the gut and pass to the liver where enzymes break them down before they reach the bloodstream. Modern technology has enabled the development of many different formulations of natural oestrogens, which remain effective in tablet form.

Oral oestradiol is rapidly converted to *oestrone* in the body. This means that if the brand of HRT contains oestradiol and oestrone, the principal active oestrogen found in the bloodstream will be oestrone. This is different from the natural pre-menopausal state, when oestradiol is the principal oestrogen. This is why some doctors argue that the oral route is unnatural; other routes of giving the hormones – skin patches and implants – enable oestradiol to enter directly into the bloodstream, unchanged.

Natural equine oestrogens
Premarin™ (Wyeth) is one of the most popular oestrogens pre-scribed. It contains natural equine oestrogens, which are similar in structure to human oestrogens. These were first refined over 60 years ago, from the urine of pregnant mares which contains large amounts of oestrogens. Because of their origin, it has been argued that these oestrogens are only natural to the horse! But doctors have prescribed *Premarin*™ as replacement therapy for over 50 years and time has proved it to be a widely used and effective treatment. However, equine oestrogens are more likely to cause side-effects of nausea and vomiting than the natural human oestrogens.

Synthetic oestrogens
Mestranol is a synthetic oestrogen that is rapidly converted in the body to another synthetic oestrogen, *ethinyloestradiol*. Synthetic oestrogens are more frequently used in the oral contraceptive pill, although occasionally ethinyloestradiol is prescribed as HRT.

Creams sometimes contain synthetic oestrogens, such as *dienoestrol* and *stilboestrol*.

Routes of giving oestrogens

Oestrogen replacement therapy comes in several different forms:

- tablet;
- patch;
- gel;
- nasal spray;
- vaginal ring;
- implant;
- vaginal cream;
- vaginal tablet;
- vaginal pessary.

Although the levels of oestrogen fluctuate widely during the menstrual cycle, the situation is quite different with hormone replacement therapy. The goal of HRT is to maintain stable levels of oestrogen, avoiding high levels that lead to side-effects such as bloating, irritability and nervousness, or low levels that would result in a return of the symptoms being treated.

Tablets

Oral oestrogen therapy is popular and has been prescribed since the 1940s. However, oral oestrogen has several important differences from the oestrogens normally produced by the ovaries:

- In pre-menopausal women, oestradiol is the dominant oestrogen circulating in the bloodstream. With oral oestrogens, oestrone is dominant.
- In pre-menopausal women, levels of oestrogen vary according to the stage of the menstrual cycle. Taking a tablet once a day causes large fluctuations in the levels of the hormones in the body. Immediately after taking a tablet, levels of oestrogen measured in the bloodstream suddenly rise, then slowly fall, until the next tablet is taken.
- Oral oestrogens are absorbed from the gut and pass straight to the liver before reaching the rest of the circulation; the liver inactivates between 30 and 90 per cent of the original dose. Most

	Advantages	*Disadvantages*
Tablets	• easy to take • easily reversible • cheap	• unnatural delivery of hormone • must be taken every day
Patches	• convenient • easy to use • more natural delivery of hormone • easily reversible	• can become detached • can irritate the skin • expensive • must be changed once or twice a week
Gel	• easy to use • more natural delivery of hormone • easily reversible	• can be messy • must cover correct amount of skin • more expensive than tablets
Nasal spray	• convenient • rapidly absorbed • perhaps fewer side-effects • easily reversible	• 'pulsed' treatment does not achieve stable levels which may be a potential problem for some conditions, e.g. migraine • expensive
Implants	• 100% compliance • more natural delivery of hormones • prolonged effect – 4 to 6 months • cheap	• needs a small surgical procedure • can cause unnaturally high levels of hormones • not easily reversible • progestogens need to be continued until no withdrawal bleed
Vaginal	• one type can be used for vaginal symptoms only, a different type is available for systemic symptoms • lasts up to 3 months • easily reversible	• additional progestogen necessary if using ring for systemic hormone absorption into the bloodstream • may cause some initial discomfort • may occasionally become dislodged
Tibolone	• easy to take • no withdrawal bleeds • easily reversible	• only for post-menopausal women • expensive

Table 1: Routes of giving oestrogens

of the break-down products are eventually removed from the body in the urine and bile. Because of this, a high oral dose is needed to enable sufficient unaltered oestrogen to reach the bloodstream, where it can be effective. This puts an unnatural load on the liver, which does not normally process such large amounts of oestrogen. Such a situation is in direct contrast to the natural process, when oestrogens from the ovaries are first diluted in the bloodstream, and much lower levels reach the liver.

- There is an enormous variation in the amount of oestrogen absorbed from tablets by different individuals. This means that two women taking the same dose of oral oestrogen may have completely different levels of oestrogen in the bloodstream.
- The necessary high dose is probably the cause of many of the side-effects of oral oestrogen therapy.

There are benefits:

- Oral oestrogens stimulate certain changes in the liver; one of these changes is the production of the high density lipoproteins (HDL), believed to help protect against heart disease. At present, it is not clear how much these liver changes are specifically due to oral therapy per se. It is possible that restoring the oestrogen in the circulation to pre-menopausal levels, by any route, is more important.

Long-term research is studying these problems but the results of small studies are encouraging. Because of this, scientists have developed different ways of giving oestrogens – implants, skin patches or gels, and vaginal creams. These routes by-pass the liver as the oestrogen is absorbed directly into the bloodstream. They also allow the levels of oestrogen to remain more constant throughout the day.

Transdermal skin patches
Giving drugs through the skin – 'transdermal' – is not a new idea: Babylonian clay tablets from around 600 BC give recipes for extracts of herbs mixed with oil and honey that were then rubbed on to the stomach of the patient as a cure for colic.

In a similar way, patches have been developed for hormone replacement, and are becoming increasingly popular. The oestrogen patch is about the size of an old ten-pence piece and looks similar to a translucent sticking plaster. A reservoir contains the supply of oestradiol. The hormones constantly pass from the patch, through the skin, into the bloodstream, over several days. The usual regimen is to change the patch on the same day twice a week – every Tuesday and Saturday, for example. There are also patches that need changing only once a week.

There are several advantages of transdermal patches over oral HRT:

- The oestrogen does not have to pass through the liver before it can be effective so the patches produce higher levels of oestrogen in the bloodstream for a lower given dose.
- Because the oestrogen is not absorbed from the gut, oestradiol is unchanged and remains the active oestrogen. This is more like the pre-menopausal situation.
- The lower dose means that there are fewer side-effects.
- Like implants, patches are particularly useful for women who have difficulty swallowing pills or who feel nauseous with oral oestrogens.
- More constant levels of oestrogen are maintained throughout the day.

Disadvantages:

- Skin reactions are an occasional problem, usually just mild itching or redness. This can be minimized by sticking the patches on a different site each time they are changed. The patch can be used on any part of the body below the waistline, usually the thigh or buttock. The buttock is probably the best place; if you are wearing a swimming costume or bikini, no one will see the patch. Never stick the patches on or near the breasts as they may enlarge. Try not to stick the patch on skin where you have used talcum powder or perfume. Occasionally some women are sensitive to the alcohol on the surface of the old-style 'reservoir' patches, e.g. Estracombi, Estraderm; removing the patch from its backing strip and leaving the alcohol to evaporate for fifteen to twenty seconds is usually effective. Fewer women have problems with the newer 'matrix' patches which look just like thin clear plastic.
- The patches usually stick very well, and you can bathe and shower as normal. However, you might have a problem if you take a lot of exercise – perspiration and frequent showering can make it

hard for the patch to stick. In these situations, you can remove the patch and put it back on to its backing strip for a few hours before reapplying it.

- Doctors are not yet certain that patches and implants are as effective as oral therapy against heart disease, because early studies on HRT and heart disease all used oral oestrogens.

- There is another potential hazard of skin patches: the *British Medical Journal* reported an incident when a patch shifted itself from the wife's thigh to her husband's back, during the night. The husband began to feel rather odd, but the explanation for his strange symptoms did not become apparent for several days!

Gel

The oestrogen gel also works by absorption of the hormone directly through the skin but, instead of using a patch as a reservoir, oestrogen is applied to the surface of the skin every day. The usual amount needed is two metered doses daily. This is best applied to the upper arm and shoulder, one dose either side, or to the thighs.

The gel is easy to use with few side-effects and the dose can be adjusted easily by the individual.

However, some women find it messy. It is also more time-consuming to use than most other methods as you should wait several minutes for the gel to dry after application.

Nasal spray

Oestrogen can also be absorbed through the skin lining the nasal passages, delivering a pulse of oestrogen rapidly into the blood-stream.

The nasal spray is effective and convenient to use, although pulsed treatment may not suit all women.

Vaginal ring

Vaginal oestrogens are usually recommended when local symptoms are the only problem, but a new vaginal ring has been developed that enables oestrogens to be absorbed through the lining of the vagina into the bloodstream. This will also effectively treat hot flushes and sweats.

The main advantages are that it is easy to use with few side-effects and can be removed for intercourse.

However, some women note initial discomfort, although this usually settles with time. The ring may become dislodged when coughing or straining.

Implants

Pellets containing oestradiol can be implanted under the skin during a routine visit to the hospital. The implant will last for about six months before it needs to be replaced. Insertion of an implant requires a small surgical procedure: a local anaesthetic is injected into the skin of the stomach, buttocks or thigh and a pellet is inserted just under the surface of the skin.

The main advantage of implant treatment is that you do not have to remember to take tablets every day or to change the patches. No one will know you are on hormone replacement therapy, and if you go on holiday there is no problem remembering treatment, unless you are away for longer than six months from the time the implant was inserted. On the negative side, it is difficult to stop therapy immediately as the implants are difficult to remove.

This method keeps the levels of oestrogen relatively constant for about four to six months, but repeated implants can occasionally lead to a build-up of unnaturally high levels. This results in all the symptoms of too much oestrogen – breast tenderness, bloatedness and nausea. Paradoxically, menopausal symptoms can reappear when the levels of oestrogen fall, even though they are still within the normal range. The implants are effective for increasingly shorter periods of time: in some cases, only a few weeks. Unfortunately it may take several years after stopping treatment for the oestrogen to return to normal post-menopausal levels. Obviously, all the distressing menopausal symptoms will recur, but these can be treated with oestrogen patches.

The main disadvantage of implant treatment is that if you have a uterus you will still need to take progestogen tablets, usually for about twelve days each month. This can be difficult to remember unless you establish a pattern – for example, starting the course on the first day of every month. If you then decide to stop implant treatment, you still have to continue the monthly progestogen until there is no withdrawal bleeding, which may take many months, even two or three years. This is because the residual effects of the implant can stimulate the lining of the uterus to thicken, increasing the risk of cancer, long after the other effects of the implant have worn off.

Vaginal creams, tablets and pessaries

Various vaginal preparations containing either natural or synthetic oestrogens are marketed in the UK.

Some preparations use oestrogens that are readily absorbed into the bloodstream from the vagina and, if these are used daily, the blood levels of oestrogen may rise sufficiently to treat hot flushes and night sweats. Regular progestogen therapy is necessary for women using these vaginal preparations which are absorbed into the bloodstream for long periods, to prevent the risk of cancer of the uterus. Fortunately, most of the creams and vaginal tablets used now to treat local symptoms have little systemic absorption so additional progestogens are rarely necessary. Because of this, they are most useful for women who are experiencing painful intercourse but who do not have any other menopausal symptoms. They help relieve any vaginal or bladder problems that are due to oestrogen deficiency, such as incontinence or repeated infections. Creams and pessaries can be messy, although this is less of a problem with the vaginal tablet. It is important not to use creams as a lubricant for intercourse; at least one case has been recorded of a man absorbing sufficient oestrogen through the skin of his penis that he started to develop breasts!

How much oestrogen do you need?

The amount of oestrogen needed differs for different women, and on the reasons for using it. The ideal dose is the lowest necessary to stop the hot flushes and other symptoms, without causing any unpleasant side-effects.

This has to be balanced against the dose that is sufficient to prevent osteoporosis, which is generally considered to be the daily equivalent of:

- 0.3–0.625 mg of oral conjugated oestrogens;
- 1–2 mg oestradiol valerate;
- 25–50 micrograms transdermal oestradiol;
- 1–5g oestrogen gel depending on the preparation.

(See Appendix 3, p. 129, for brand names.)

Unfortunately, all these doses stimulate the lining of the uterus to thicken, increasing the risk of cancer. If lower doses are used, the protection against osteoporosis and heart disease is lost.

Any doctor prescribing HRT will try to tailor the treatment

according to your individual requirements and preferences. It is useful to make a note of any problems or side-effects you notice after starting HRT, such as any bleeding or spotting, feeling sick, etc., to discuss with the doctor. It might be necessary to make some changes to the dose or type of HRT you take.

Progestogens

The main reason for adding progestogen to oestrogen replacement therapy is to create regular bleeding and to prevent cancer. You do not need to take progestogens if you have had a hysterectomy.

Using the same classification as oestrogens, progestogens can be grouped into *natural* and *synthetic* preparations. The only natural progestogen is progesterone. All other progestogens are synthetic, i.e. their chemical structure is dissimilar to that of the natural hormone.

Natural progesterone

Oral progesterone is available but, like natural oestrogens, the liver inactivates much of it before it reaches the rest of the body. This would make it necessary to take quite high doses, at least twice a day, to enable sufficient active progesterone into the circulation. Unfortunately, this also increases side-effects: acne, weight gain, water retention, breast discomfort and pre-menstrual symptoms. Drowsiness is a particular problem with oral progesterone, so the highest dose is taken at bedtime.

Progesterone suppositories are sometimes prescribed, but it is not a popular treatment in the UK. More of the hormone reaches the circulation than by the oral route, and treatment is only necessary once a day. The suppositories can be inserted either into the rectum or into the vagina. More popular is the recently developed vaginal gel, which is used on alternate days.

There has been a great deal of interest in progesterone cream derived from plant sources, typically the Mexican wild yam. Although anecdotal reports seem promising, at the time of writing there are no well-designed studies to confirm claims of benefits.

Synthetic progestogens

Because of the problems of absorption, most of the progesterone used for hormone replacement therapy is synthetic. There are two main groups of synthetic progestogens: progestogens that have a chemical structure similar to the natural progesterone, and progestogens structurally related to the male hormone, testosterone.

Progestogens derived from progesterone:

- dydrogesterone;
- medroxyprogesterone.

Progestogens derived from testosterone are more likely to cause acne and greasy hair and skin than the progesterone analogues:

- norgestrel;
- levonorgestrel;
- norethisterone.

A new generation of progestogens are available. These are believed to have fewer side-effects but, unfortunately, although used for contraception, they are not yet available for use as HRT:

- desogestrel;
- norgestimate;
- gestodene;
- drospirenone.

A large percentage of women, up to 20 to 30 per cent, notice additional side-effects – breast tenderness, nausea, depression, irritability, headaches and water retention – during the latter part of the progestogen course. These are much like the symptoms of premenstrual syndrome. Usually, lowering the dose or changing the type of progestogen can relieve some of these symptoms.

Routes of giving progestogens

There are several ways of administering progestogen:

- tablets;
- transdermal patches;
- vaginal gel;
- intra-uterine system;
- pessaries/suppositories.

Tablets

This is the commonest form of treatment with progestogen. Synthetic progestogens are usually given, but natural progesterone is available in tablet form for hormone replacement therapy.

Transdermal skin patches

Until recently, progestogens were only available as tablets, and this meant that women using oestrogen patches still had to take a course of progestogen tablets every month. Not surprisingly, this combination of two completely different modes of drug delivery was unacceptable to some women.

One brand of double patches looks similar to a pair of goggles – although much smaller. They contain oestrogen in one patch, joined to a second patch containing progestogen. A more recent patch combines oestrogen and progestogen in a single patch that looks like thin plastic film. Unlike oral progestogen, when much of the dose is lost before it reaches the bloodstream, patches mean that lower doses of progestogen can be used, which minimizes side-effects.

Patches containing only oestrogen are changed every three or four days for the first two weeks of the cycle. For the final two weeks of the cycle the 'double' patch is used in the same way. Most women should have some bleeding towards the end of the two weeks of using the 'double' patch, usually starting on day 24 to 26 of treatment.

Vaginal gel

Natural progesterone is available as a vaginal gel and is licensed for HRT. It is generally used every couple of days for the last 12 days of the cycle followed by a monthly 'period', although in some clinical trials it has been used twice weekly together with oestrogen as part of a continuous combined regimen.

Pessaries/suppositories

Rectal and vaginal suppositories are sometimes used for women experiencing bad side-effects from progestogens but doctors rarely prescribe these as they are not licensed for HRT.

Intrauterine system

This is similar to the copper 'coil' or intra-uterine device (IUD) that is used as a highly effective contraceptive. Instead of copper, the intrauterine system has a reservoir of the progestogen levonorgestrel, which is slowly released into the bloodstream. Although this contraceptive is not, at the time of writing, licensed for use to oppose oestrogen for HRT, studies show that it can be effective when used in this way. Side-effects are much lower than with oral progestogens and the contraceptive effect can be an advantage for women whose periods have not yet ceased. The main disadvantage is irregular bleeding, usually only in the early months of use; in about 20 per cent of women, periods stop altogether within the first year.

How much progestogen do you need?

All progestogenic side-effects of depression, breast tenderness, bloating and water retention are related to the dose – higher doses result in more side-effects.

Doctors usually prescribe a low dose of progestogen initially; the minimum dosage of progestogen that is sufficient to protect against cancer of the uterus is recommended. The necessary daily oral doses taken for a minimum of 12 days a month are:

- 170 or 250 micrograms norethisterone patch;
- 1 mg oral norethisterone;
- 20 micrograms levonorgestrel patch;
- 75–250 micrograms oral levonorgestrel tablet;
- 150–500 micrograms oral norgestrel;
- 10–20 mg oral medroxyprogesterone acetate;
- 10–20 mg oral dydrogesterone;
- 4% gel alternate days vaginal progesterone.

The amount required for continuous progestogen (taken every day) is different:

- 0.5–1 mg norethisterone tablet;
- 170 micrograms norethisterone patch;
- 2.5–5 mg medroxyprogesterone acetate tablet;
- 5 mg dydrogesterone tablet.

(See Appendix 3, p. 129, for brand names.)

Some doctors increase the dose if withdrawal bleeding regularly occurs before the eleventh day of the progestogen course, until the dose is sufficient to delay the start of bleeding until day 12 or later.

Tibolone: Livial™ (Organon)

Tibolone is a synthetic steroid that has the combined actions of oestrogens, androgens and progestogens. Your doctor can prescribe it for the treatment of post-menopausal symptoms following either natural menopause or surgical removal of the ovaries.

It is taken every day with no drug-free interval. Because it has combined effects, an additional monthly course of progestogens is unnecessary. The main advantage of tibolone is that there is no withdrawal bleeding. However, unpredictable irregular bleeding can be a problem, particularly if it is taken within a year of your last period, or you change to tibolone directly from oestrogen replacement therapy. Because of this, women should not use tibolone unless they have not had a natural period for at least a year.

Like standard oestrogen replacement therapy, tibolone treats hot flushes and night sweats. It also improves vaginal lubrication, easing painful intercourse and so increases sexual enjoyment.

It can benefit libido and is also licensed for osteoporosis. The risk of heart disease does not appear to be affected, but long-term studies are necessary to determine the true effects. At present, it is not recommended for women who have heart disease or thrombosis, so it is not an alternative for women who are unable to take HRT for medical reasons.

Testosterone

Implants of the male sex hormone testosterone are sometimes prescribed in addition to oestrogen. The adrenal gland normally produces testosterone in women, albeit at much lower levels than in men. This hormone seems to be important in maintaining the sex drive. As women age, they produce less testosterone, so replacement of this hormone may help restore libido.

It can cause voice changes and unwanted hair growth, particularly if the dose is too high.

Testosterone is currently only available as an implant but patches and gels are being evaluated.

How do you decide which route to use?

- Oral therapy has stood the test of time and is a good choice if you can easily remember to take tablets every day.
- Patches, gels, the nasal spray, the systemic vaginal ring or implants are best if you do not absorb the tablets, or the oestrogen tablets make you feel nauseous. Women who have high blood pressure or liver problems are also advised to use a non-oral route.

- Gels, the nasal spray or the systemic vaginal ring are useful if you cannot take tablets and patches irritate the skin.
- Implants are best for women who have had a hysterectomy as otherwise it is still necessary to take a monthly course of progestogen.
- Local vaginal preparations can be used if vaginal symptoms are the only problem.

Different regimens

This section of the chapter discusses the various options available, and the disadvantages and advantages of each regimen. There are several different regimens to choose between, but it mostly depends on whether you still have a uterus.

Sometimes it is necessary to try a few different regimens before finding the most suitable:

My GP first put me on a cyclical dose of HRT – a combination pack. This took away the flushes and sweats, but increased the depression, and gave me sore, swollen breasts.

My GP suggested that we try and sort out a suitable dosage of HRT by combining the progestogen, norethisterone, with the oestrogen patches. A dosage of 50-microgram patches, twice weekly for three weeks, plus 5 mg norethisterone from day 12 to day 24 of my cycle certainly helped. However, when starting the progestogen on day 12, my period would often come as early as day 18 or 19. Three weeks between the beginning of each period became normal. The sweats and flushes only came during the week without oestrogen and the depression lifted, although the PMT symptoms remained. We increased the dosage of oestrogen to 100 micrograms to try and alleviate the remaining symptoms. This proved too much, with the depression and insomnia returning.

Further reading gave me the idea that I could be taking oestrogen for the whole month. I discussed this with my GP. I also realized that after taking the progestogen for five days, my PMT symptoms appeared. My GP is sympathetic and after further experiments I now use oestrogen patches 50 microgram twice a week, every week, and norethisterone 5 mg for seven days, every fourth week.

If you have had a hysterectomy

Women who have had a hysterectomy can take oestrogen alone. Some of the older regimens advocated that the oestrogen was taken for three weeks, followed by a one-week break, before starting the cycle again. The aim of this was to simulate the menstrual cycle, but there is no advantage to this. Furthermore, the menopausal symptoms can return during the seven-day interval. To this end, the current recommendation is to maintain constant levels of oestrogen by taking daily tablets, once- or twice-weekly skin patches, or six-monthly implants.

Women who have not had a hysterectomy

Women who still have a uterus have the added complication of needing progestogen to protect against cancer of the uterus.

This involves several choices:

1 choice of regimen: e.g. continuous or cyclic;
2 route of drug: e.g. tablets or patches.

Choice of regimen

- Continuous oestrogen and cyclical progestogen, i.e. oestrogen taken daily without a break combined with a course of progestogen each month.
- Continuous oestrogen and continuous progestogen, i.e. both hormones taken daily without a break.

Cyclical combinations

Various schedules have been advocated for cyclical combined therapy with both oestrogens and progestogens.

In the UK, most women take oestrogens continuously, without a break, adding progestogen tablets for around 12 days of each 28-day treatment cycle. Various regimens are available: some have been designed to mimic the oestrogen fluctuations of the normal menstrual cycle.

Some doctors prescribe 25 days of oestrogen per cycle, adding progestogens on the last 12 days of each oestrogen cycle. Other regimens favour a week free from treatment every month, but symptoms can return during this break. Both these regimens have fallen out of favour since the advantages of continuous oestrogens have been recognized.

Whatever the regimen, most women have some vaginal bleeding, similar to a period, near the end of the progestogen course. This is because the progestogens have the effect of expelling the lining of the uterus. Unlike normal menstruation, this withdrawal bleeding is not an indicator of fertility, as the ovaries do not release an egg. The bleeding is usually light, lasting four to five days.

About 10 to 15 per cent of women do not have any bleeding while on a regimen of cyclical oestrogen/progestogen. This is quite normal and does not mean that the HRT is not effective – it is just that the endometrium has not thickened so there is nothing to be removed.

Continuous combinations
The unfortunate main side-effect of progestogen is the withdrawal bleeding. This leads many women to stop HRT. The aim of continuous combined therapy is to eliminate monthly bleeding. Oestrogen therapy stimulates the endometrium, the lining of the uterus. The theory is that if progestogen is taken daily, it can prevent any development of the endometrium and the subsequent risk of cancer. Since there is no lining to shed, there is no bleeding.

However, about 80 per cent of women taking continuous combined therapy experience some initial irregular bleeding, usually because this type of HRT is started too soon, before a woman's own hormones have died down. For this reason, continuous combined HRT is only recommended for women who have been post-menopausal for at least one year, or after the age of 54 if women have continued with cyclical HRT.

Some studies show that starting treatment with a lower dose of oestrogen and a higher dose of progestogen can prevent any initial bleeding. The dose can be altered later, increasing the dose of oestrogen to maximize its effects, and reducing the progestogen to minimize side-effects. However, some women may experience irregular bleeding for the first time after several months of treatment.

Side-effects of continuous progestogens are variable: some researchers report appreciable problems with breast tenderness, irritability, headaches and depression; other researchers report these symptoms to be fewer than with cyclical regimens.

This method of HRT does seem effective in reducing the oestrogen stimulus to the uterus; biopsies from women who do not bleed on this regimen have shown minimal thickening of the uterine lining.

There are possible added benefits in that continuous progestogen may stimulate bone formation, acting in synergism with oestrogen to prevent osteoporosis.

Route of administration
The combinations most commonly prescribed are:

- oral oestrogen plus oral progestogen;
- oestrogen patches plus oral progestogen;
- oestrogen and progestogen combined patches.

Oestrogen gel, nasal spray or systemic vaginal ring can also be used together with oral progestogen or vaginal progesterone.

The advantages and disadvantages of each are discussed earlier in the chapter. Unless there are medical reasons why you need to use a particular route of treatment, the choice depends on whether you can remember to take tablets every day. A greater problem is remembering the course of progestogen tablets each month. This is more difficult if you are using oestrogen skin patches or implants than if you are already taking oral oestrogen.

Because the progestogen is so important, some drug companies have produced calendar packs. These are designed to make it easier to remember when to take each hormone.

The main disadvantage of the calendar packs is that the type and dose of the progestogen is fixed. Prescribing the oestrogen and the progestogen separately enables the dose of each hormone to be adjusted as necessary, to minimize side-effects. It is possible to occasionally alter the time of the bleeding by delaying the course of progestogen, or taking it earlier. This is useful if the bleeding is timed to coincide with a holiday or other special event. But prescribing the hormones separately returns the problem of remembering when to take the course of progestogen. One method is to take the progestogen for the first 12 to 14 days of every calendar month. This has the advantage of being an easy-to-follow regimen. Also, all bleeding will occur around the middle of the month. This makes it easier for you and your doctor to notice unusual bleeding patterns that might need further investigation. It is not wise to take shorter courses than the usually recommended 12 to 14 days, as it is more likely to cause irregular bleeding and increases the risk of cancer.

Some specialists feel that a 14-day course of progestogens every three months gives sufficient protection from cancer of the endometrium. This is a particular advantage for women whose periods have become very irregular but for whom it is too early to start a no-bleed regimen.

Can women with a uterus take oestrogens without progestogen?

Early HRT regimens advocated taking oestrogen on its own for three weeks, followed by a week free from treatment. The aim was that in women with an intact uterus, a 'period' would occur during this free week, discharging any thickening of the lining of the uterus that had built up. Research has shown that this does not always happen, and there is a risk of the thickened lining turning cancerous. Fortunately, the type of cancer of the uterus that usually develops when taking HRT is very specific and responds well to treatment.

Even though the risk of this type of cancer is small, doctors advise every woman with a uterus to take progestogen in addition to oestrogen. But many women find it hard to tolerate the effects of progestogen, especially the monthly bleeding. This is particularly relevant for older post-menopausal women, who are least likely to put up with a withdrawal bleed but who may have osteoporosis, suffer painful intercourse or have urinary problems.

However, the dangers of unopposed oestrogens are well documented and the decision to take oestrogens alone should be made with the full knowledge of the increased risks. To check that cancer is not developing, these women should have a biopsy at least once a year. This used to involve taking a small piece of tissue from the uterus, usually requiring a D and C operation and an overnight stay in hospital. Nowadays a small sample can be taken in the outpatient department, either by a procedure similar to fitting a contraceptive coil or, more often now, during a hysteroscopy during which a camera is inserted into the womb. Although it can cause some immediate discomfort, it is much less unpleasant than a D and C.

The greatest problem is the increased long-term risk of cancer of the uterus, even after stopping oestrogen replacement. One study found that the increased risk remained for as long as ten years, after only twelve months of oestrogen therapy. This is particularly the case after treatment with implants of oestrogen – some doctors recommend that women who decide to stop implant therapy should continue with regular courses of progestogens, every month, until they stop having withdrawal bleeding.

The cost of HRT

Appendix 3, p. 129, lists some of the different brands of hormone replacement therapy currently available.

All the types of HRT discussed in this chapter are available on the NHS. Oestrogen therapy carries a single prescription charge. Any combination of oestrogen and progestogen in a cyclical regimen carries a double prescription charge. However, the continuous combined therapy, despite containing both oestrogen and progestogen, only carries a single prescription charge. Tibolone also carries a single prescription charge.

These charges do not reflect the true cost of the treatment, and if you pay for a private prescription the cost will vary depending on the type and dose of HRT prescribed. The conjugated oestrogens are the cheapest available form of oestrogen (at the time of writing, monthly cost £3.24 for the daily 0.625 mg dose). The cost of a 12–14 day course of progestogen is £1.05 for 10 mg dydrogesterone but £11.08 for Crinone vaginal gel.

Oestrogen patches are more expensive than oral HRT. A month's supply of oestrogen patches currently costs between £4.56 and £7.03 for the standard 50 microgram dose. If the combined oestrogen/progestogen patches are used for two weeks, the total monthly cost of the patch treatment is around £10.

Tibolone is the most expensive from of HRT: the monthly cost is £13.05.

Summary

- Hormone replacement therapy is available as tablets, patches, gels, a nasal spray, implants and vaginal preparations.
- Unless you have had a hysterectomy, you need regular courses of progestogen therapy to prevent the small but significant risk of cancer of the uterus.
- If you have had a hysterectomy, you can take oestrogen on its own – there is no need for progestogen.
- Regimens vary. The commonest regimen is to take oestrogen daily, without a break. If progestogens are necessary, they are taken for a minimum of seven days every month. A 12 to 14 day course is safer.
- Calendar packs of oestrogen and progestogen are available to aid

compliance. Alternatively, the course of progestogen tablets can be started on the first day of every calendar month.

- Patches containing oestrogen and progestogen obviate the need for a course of oral progestogen as the combined patches are used for two weeks of the four-week cycle.
- On all regimens using cyclical progestogens, withdrawal bleeding usually occurs near the end of the progestogen course. This is an artificial 'period' and does not indicate fertility.
- Alternatively, progestogens can be taken in combination with oestrogen, every day without interruption, starting after the menopause. This can cause irregular bleeding in the early days, particularly if started too close to the menopause. Most women will eventually have no bleeding at all. The daily dose of progestogen adequately protects the uterus.
- The minimum effective dose of the hormones is usually pre-scribed, sufficient to prevent osteoporosis as well as alleviating other menopausal symptoms.
- Tibolone is a synthetic hormone for women starting HRT after the menopause. Additional progestogens are not needed, so there is no regular monthly bleeding.

8

Beyond the Menopause

Making the decision whether or not to take HRT is not always easy, and there are more choices to make if you decide to go ahead. Many women stop treatment too soon, unaware of the commitment necessary to achieve maximum benefit from treatment. There are numerous reasons why a woman stops treatment: side-effects or fear of the potential risks, lack of expected effects, or just forgetting to take it. Probably most of the reasons stem from an initial lack of information about HRT, certainly about the long-term benefits. Not everyone taking HRT finds that it suits them, but simple adjustments to the dose or hormones or changing to a different regime may be sufficient to enable you to continue treatment.

Having started treatment, the next question is: how long should you take it for? The answer depends largely on the reasons why you initiated treatment, usually falling into one of two categories:

- *Short-term treatment* for relief of menopausal symptoms – usually the benefits are obvious as the symptoms are noticeably relieved.
- *Long-term treatment* for prevention of osteoporosis – this requires a greater commitment: the benefits are not obvious as you are taking treatment to prevent a condition that may not give rise to any symptoms.

Duration of treatment for short-term relief

The most common reason for taking HRT is to relieve symptoms. Many of these symptoms – the hot flushes, night sweats, palpitations, irritability, poor concentration and depression – start before the periods cease. They are self-limiting and die out within a couple of years or so for the majority of women, so less than five years is considered sufficient duration of treatment for menopausal symptoms. The HRT is then tailed off gradually over two to three months. If it is stopped too quickly, the hot flushes and night sweats can return.

Sometimes the symptoms are as severe as before treatment started. If so, it may be necessary to restart the HRT and continue for a few months longer before tailing the treatment off again. Up to 25 per cent of women continue to have menopausal symptoms for up to five years, so may need to take HRT for this length of time, until the symptoms abate. Unfortunately there is no way of predicting who will need longer-term treatment; it is necessary to tail off the HRT at intervals to assess the response.

It is not unusual for symptoms of vaginal dryness and painful intercourse to become a problem after stopping treatment with HRT, even if the hot flushes and night sweats have ceased. These symptoms respond well to oestrogen creams, tablets or pessaries inserted into the vagina using a special applicator. A vaginal ring that is effective for up to three months is also available

Duration of treatment for long-term prevention

It is not easy to take treatment for any length of time, and even more so if its effects are not that obvious: the effects of osteoporosis may not be apparent for many years after the menopause. Yet there is strong evidence that if you are happy to take HRT, its continued use is associated with a reduced risk of fractures. This can mean a better quality of life and increased life expectancy. In general, treatment to prevent osteoporosis needs to be for at least five years, started soon after the menopause, if not lifelong.

Few doctors refuse to prescribe treatment if a patient requests it (only 0.2 per cent in one study), although obviously they will only prescribe HRT if you are suitable for it. Even then, the alternatives are still worth considering.

Short-term or long-term?

Obviously the choice is not always going to be straightforward. Some women may start treatment for symptomatic relief, and for various reasons decide to continue. Others may initiate therapy with the idea of taking it for several years and then find they are unable to tolerate side-effects. If in doubt, always discuss these problems with your GP or a doctor at a specialist clinic. There are few hard and fast rules about HRT and there may be ways of overcoming the perceived problem. Furthermore, the field of knowledge about HRT is continually expanding, as the results of further research become available.

When is the best time to start HRT?

The best time to start HRT is when your periods are irregular or have just stopped. Women who had an artificial menopause by having their ovaries removed or treated with radiotherapy should start HRT immediately. Therapy is more effective the closer it is initiated to the menopause, because it is impossible to restore any significant amount of bone once it has been lost.

Can women start taking HRT after the menopause?

Although there is no upper age limit for starting treatment with HRT, some doctors are reticent to initiate therapy to women years after the menopause. In one study, 96 per cent of doctors would prescribe HRT before the periods have stopped completely for the relief of symptoms. In contrast, about 30 per cent of doctors were prepared to prescribe HRT up to ten years after the menopause, but only 23 per cent would consider starting treatment more than ten years after periods had stopped.

But there is a strong argument for treating post-menopausal women who have never taken oestrogen in the past. Oestrogen replacement can reverse some of the changes even if it is not begun until years after the menopause; it can help restore the vaginal secretions years after pain and bleeding have prevented a woman enjoying intercourse.

The effects on osteoporosis are also significant: one study showed that when a group of women aged between 65 and 74 were given oestrogen, they had fewer hip fractures. In addition, if a woman has already fractured a bone, HRT will reduce the risk of further fractures. There is accumulating evidence that oestrogen, with or without progestogen, appears to be effective therapy even in women with established osteoporosis.

Older women taking oestrogen replacement for the first time several years after the menopause usually need a lower dose of oestrogen than women starting it at the time of the menopause.

How long can you take HRT for?

There is no evidence that HRT has to be stopped at any age, and treatment can continue for as long as it is necessary, even for the rest of your life. The major concern about long-term use is the possible increased risk of breast cancer but the evidence is conflicting.

A few women have taken HRT for more than thirty years, for its continued protection against heart disease and osteoporosis; when HRT is discontinued, bone loss resumes as it would have done after the natural menopause. It used to be thought that there was a greater loss of bone after stopping hormone replacement therapy, but more recent evidence suggests that the rate of bone loss is equivalent to the rate that normally follows the menopause.

Summary

- The length of time you should take HRT depends on why you take it. For the symptomatic treatment of the menopause, you need to take it for between two and three years at least, tailing the dose down slowly at the end.
- For the prevention of osteoporosis, a minimum of five years is recommended, but lifelong if possible.
- The optimum time to start HRT is around the time of the menopause, but starting it later in life is still associated with many benefits.

9

Where to Go for Advice

Reading a book about the menopause and hormone replacement therapy can only give you a limited amount of information. Books can give an overview but may not contain the answers to your specific problems.

Most women in the UK consult their general practitioner. The majority of GPs are sympathetic but the recent advances in menopause research and therapy make it difficult for doctors to keep up to date, unless they have a particular interest in the subject. Neither is a busy GP surgery the ideal place to discuss the pros and cons of treatment, let alone the alternatives, since the average consultation lasts only 5.2 minutes.

If you have a local well woman or family planning clinic, it is worthwhile seeking their help. You can also contact the gynaecology department of your local hospital – a few now have a special menopause clinic. There are also several private clinics. For a list of clinics in your area (private and NHS), look in your local telephone directory or contact the Family Planning Association (FPA) Head-quarters, 2–12 Pentonville Road, London N1 9FP (see Appendix 2, p. 127).

If you live in London or the South East, you can visit the Amarant Clinic, a not-for-profit clinic that deals exclusively with the treatment of the menopause – see later in this chapter.

Most NHS clinics and even private clinics require a referral letter from your GP. This may seem a nuisance, particularly if your GP is against the idea. However, if you are ever taken ill as an emergency, it is important that your GP knows exactly which treatments you are taking, so it is always better to keep your GP informed.

Your GP

If you have menopausal symptoms or you are interested in HRT, go to your family doctor first. If you decide to go ahead with treatment, your GP can prescribe this on the NHS, at the cost of a standard prescription fee.

Your GP may prefer to refer you to a gynaecology outpatient

clinic at your local hospital. An increasing number of GPs now run their own well woman and menopause clinics, as a separate service from the routine surgery, so that they will have more time to discuss the different options available.

NHS menopause clinics

You usually have to be referred by your GP before you can be seen at a hospital clinic. Some of the larger teaching hospital clinics are also research centres, so you might be asked to help with some of the clinical trials that are underway; these help doctors to improve the treatments available. It is your right to refuse to enter a clinical trial and a refusal should not affect your treatment in any way. All trials are carefully screened to check that they are as safe as current knowledge permits. They must follow strict guidelines and the trial has to be passed by the local Ethical Committee before any patients can take part. You cannot be included in any trial without your permission. The doctors undertaking the trial should be happy to answer your questions.

Since the doctors at the clinic may not have all the information that your GP has regarding your general health, you will be asked questions about your medical history, and the doctor will also give you a full medical examination, including an internal examination. You will then be given a trial of HRT, if indicated. At the follow-up visit the doctor will make any necessary adjustments to the treatment. You should mention any problems you have had, however trivial. If you have had unexplained irregular bleeding, the doctor may suggest that the lining of the womb is checked with a biopsy or hysteroscopy. This is often done in the outpatient department, but occasionally you may need to stay at the hospital overnight.

If, at the second visit, you are happy with the treatment, you will be asked to return for follow-up visits at the hospital, usually six-monthly or annually. You may prefer to see your GP for further prescriptions, but you can always make an appointment to return to the hospital clinic if necessary.

Private clinics

Private clinics essentially run in a similar fashion to a hospital outpatient department, although the waiting list is usually minimal. You will have to pay a fee, although it might be possible to use private health insurance to cover the costs. Although a referral letter from your GP is not essential, it is preferred. In any case, the doctor at the clinic will usually send a report of the consultation to your GP.

The Amarant Trust

The Amarant Trust is a charity set up in 1986 by Teresa Gorman MP and Malcolm Whitehead, a leading expert in HRT. The aims of the Trust are to promote a better understanding of the menopause, to support and expand research in the field, and to make information and treatment available to all women. The doctors who run the clinic have up-to-date knowledge of all the treatments available and can offer impartial advice to help you choose the most suitable treatment. They are concerned about all aspects of the menopause, not just HRT. The clinic also offers additional tests such as cervical smears, mammograms, thyroid function tests, etc.

In addition to running a specialist menopause clinic the Amarant Trust offers a free Helpline (01293 413000, standard rate call charge), prerecorded Adviceline tapes (09068 660620, premium rate call charge) and a selection of leaflets and publications. The Helpline is manned by a team of nurses who can provide information on any query relating to the menopause and HRT. Lines are open weekdays from 11 a.m. to 6 p.m.

The Amarant Trust provides the names and addresses of menopause and HRT clinics all over the UK. An information pack costs £6, but for £20 you can become a 'Friend' of the Amarant Trust, which entitles you to receive all the Amarant publications, updated leaflets and any other information updates. The address is listed under 'Useful Addresses' in Appendix 2, p. 127.

What happens at a menopause clinic?

The first visit

A series of routine checks may be undertaken.
  You might be asked about:

- any menopausal symptoms;
- the date of your last period;
- your menstrual pattern, contraception, and any pregnancies;

- your present and past health;
- your family's health, and whether any blood relatives have angina or heart attacks, strokes, blood clots (thrombosis), breast cancer, or fractures;
- how much alcohol you drink;
- what medicines you take regularly, or have taken in the past;
- whether or not you smoke, or used to smoke;
- how much exercise you take and your usual diet.

The following tests may be done:

- blood pressure;
- height;
- weight;
- breast examination and mammogram, if indicated;
- internal examination and smear test, if indicated;
- urine test, to check for infections and diabetes;
- very occasionally, a blood test is necessary to confirm the diagnosis of the menopause, or separate tests to measure cholesterol levels or risk of blood clots (thrombophilia screen).

If the results of these tests are satisfactory, the doctor will discuss the different forms of HRT with you, and answer any questions you might have. If you are interested in any alternatives to HRT, now is the time to mention it.

If you decide to try HRT, the doctor will prescribe one brand and ask you to return after trying it for about three months. You may be given a 'bleeding chart' on which you should record any spotting or bleeding that occurs during treatment. You should also make a note of any other symptoms you experience. Ask the doctor who you should contact if you have any problems before your next appointment.

The most common problems early in treatment are usually:

- *Side-effects of treatment* Typical side-effects include nausea, breast tenderness and leg cramps. These are to be expected and usually resolve spontaneously after a few weeks.
- *Irregular bleeding* Breakthrough bleeding is not unusual at the start of therapy. It is usually light, lasting no more than a couple of days. It should resolve within the first six months of treatment.
- *Menopausal symptoms are not fully controlled* Most women notice an improvement in their symptoms within the first few

weeks but maximum benefit may not be achieved until three months.

It is important to be aware of this early 'settling down' period as many women stop treatment before it has had a chance to be effective. You cannot accurately assess your response to HRT until you have taken it for at least three months. If you are still having problems after this time, these can often be controlled by simple adjustments to the dose or type of hormones taken. If that particular type of HRT did not suit you, an alternative type may be recommended.

Once the most suitable form is decided upon, you usually return to the clinic every six to twelve months for a check-up. You can choose to see your GP instead.

Follow-up visits

At these visits, you may be seen by the clinic nurse, who can refer you to the doctor if there are any problems. The nurse will check your height, weight and blood pressure, and ask you a few questions. You should tell the nurse or doctor if you have had any of the following problems:

- unusual vaginal bleeding or discharge;
- unexpected weight gain;
- headaches or migraines;
- difficulty with vision;
- trouble with veins in the legs;
- any other problems or possible side-effects since starting the HRT.

The nurse or doctor may check your breasts or arrange a mammogram, if indicated. Every three to five years, you will also have an internal examination and cervical smear test until you reach the age of 65.

Screening for problems

Prevention is an important aspect of medicine – it is much easier to treat diseases early than it is to treat them later. Screening programmes are an important part of prevention. Your doctor will routinely check for high blood pressure, breast lumps and cervical cancer as part of the national screening programme.

Breast checks

Many women have naturally lumpy breasts and find it difficult to check their breasts for lumps. However, if you check them every month, you will soon learn what is normal for you. Look for any lumps or unusual changes, such as discharge from the nipple. Do not check your breasts just before a period as they naturally enlarge and become swollen at this time; the best time is just after your period.

The breast test

- Stand in front of a mirror, arms hanging relaxed by your sides. Look at your breasts in the mirror – are there any obvious differences, does the skin look puckered anywhere, has the nipple become inverted, or is there a discharge? Look for any rashes or discoloration of the skin.
- Next, rest your hands on your hips, pressing firmly, looking for any differences between each breast. The skin should stay smooth, with no dimpling. Raise your straight arms above your head, again looking for any changes. Lower your arms.
- Turn to each side, and look again.
- Lying flat on the floor, support your shoulders with a flat pillow, so that your neck is slightly arched. Lift your left arm up behind your head, bent at the elbow. With your right hand, gently squeeze the left nipple, noting any discharge. Using the flat of your right hand, feel your left breast for any lumps, pressing gently over each part of the breast. Do not forget to feel the part of the breast that runs up into the armpit. Repeat again with your left arm by your side, then follow the same procedure for the right breast.
- If you do find a lump, see your doctor. It may be nothing, but no one will think you are wasting their time. It is much better to be reassured rather than worry needlessly, as many lumps are simple cysts. If it is something more serious, it is sensible to have it treated sooner rather than later.

Mammograms

The recommendation is that all post-menopausal women should have a mammogram every two to three years, usually until the age of 65 although older women can still request them. This special type of X-ray shows up abnormal changes in the breast tissue when they are very small, before they can be felt.

Cervical smear tests

Most women will have had a cervical smear test at some time before the menopause. It is now usually carried out in the UK every three to five years, on women between the ages of 20 and 65.

The standard smear test is the Papanicolau, or Pap, test – named after the Greek gynaecologist who first described the technique. The doctor or nurse will ask you to lie on your side, with your knees bent up towards your chin. The alternative is to lie on your back; bend your knees up, and then drop one to each side. A plastic or metal speculum is passed into the vagina until the cervix, which is the neck of the uterus, can be seen. The cervix is gently scraped with a spatula to remove a few of the cells, which are then smeared on to a glass slide. The slide is sent to a laboratory where it is examined under a microscope, enabling the detection of any abnormal cells.

It helps if you can try to relax; if you are tense, the vaginal muscles also tense up and it can make the insertion of the speculum painful. You may notice some slight bleeding after the test – this is entirely normal.

Other tests you might be offered

Diagnosing the menopause

In the majority of cases, the symptoms that you describe are sufficient for your doctor to confirm the menopause. There are exceptions – for example, women who have an early menopause – when the diagnosis may be in doubt. In these cases, a blood test will show low levels of oestradiol, combined with high levels of follicle stimulating hormone (FSH). This is the most reliable test for diagnosis, but it is not always possible to measure these hormones accurately, and tests are expensive.

Another method, occasionally used for women who have had a natural menopause, is the progestogen challenge test. Progestogen tablets are taken for ten days; if no bleeding occurs at the end of the progestogen course, the diagnosis of the menopause is confirmed.

Ultrasound scan

This can be useful to identify some causes of bleeding, such as fibroids or polyps, and is also used to help identify cancer of the ovaries. The method is very safe and only takes a few minutes. It is usually done by passing a probe into the vagina, while you are lying on a couch – similar to having a smear test.

Cholesterol tests
Many centres offer blood tests to check cholesterol levels. A high cholesterol count has been linked to an increased risk of strokes and heart attacks (see Chapter 5).

Bone density assessments
There are no simple screening tests for osteoporosis, and at least 25 per cent of bone must be lost before routine X-rays will detect a problem. The only reliable test currently available is to measure the thickness of the bone. This is usually done using *dual energy X-ray absorptiometry (DEXA)*. It gives a very low dose of radiation, and takes only a few minutes.

These tests are painless – unlike an X-ray, you keep your clothes on and all you have to do is relax on a couch while the machine passes over you. Most of these techniques involve a small amount of radiation.

Newer mass screening techniques using ultrasound are becoming more popular.

Summary

- Visit your GP first. Discuss your symptoms and your feelings about treatment. Ask about the alternatives to HRT. Very few GPs will refuse to prescribe HRT for the relief of menopausal symptoms, but it may be that you cannot take HRT for medical reasons or that your symptoms are due to a different problem.
- If your GP is unsympathetic, or does not have sufficient time or knowledge to discuss all the pros and cons of the different treatments available, you can ask to be referred to a hospital or private menopause clinic.
- It is occasionally possible to refer yourself, without a letter from your GP, although it is wise to let your GP know that you are doing this.
- In most cases, your symptoms are sufficient to make the diagnosis of the menopause. Tests are rarely necessary.
- If you opt for HRT, you are usually asked to try one type for a few months, before returning to the clinic to discuss any problems.
- Problems are common in the early months, maximum benefit is not achieved until three months, so persevere.

- There are many different types of HRT, and many different ways of taking it, so if you do not get on with one it is worth trying another.
- Get to know your own body – checking your breasts regularly for lumps helps you differentiate between the normal lumps and any unusual changes.
- The doctor or nurse will perform regular checks as indicated by the symptoms you experience. If you have any odd symptoms, note them down to tell the doctor. A simple change in the dose or type of treatment may be all that is needed.
- Finally, if you are not sure about something – ask!

10

The Alternatives

Hormone replacement therapy is not the only option available for women experiencing menopausal symptoms; some women do not want to take hormones, some are advised not to take HRT for medical reasons, and others stop HRT because of side-effects.

This chapter discusses some of the alternatives to HRT as well as self-help approaches. The final section gives advice on exercise for a healthy heart and strong bones.

Symptom relief

Hot flushes

Self-help
Simple ways of keeping cool can reduce the intensity of hot flushes.

- Wear natural fabrics next to the skin rather than synthetic.
- Layer your clothes so that if you suddenly get too hot, you can easily remove a sweater or cardigan.
- Avoid nylon sheets – natural fabrics breathe and will be much more comfortable.
- Give up cigarettes, alcohol and coffee – particularly late at night. These affect blood vessels and make you more prone to flushing.
- Oil of evening primrose may help pre-menstrual symptoms as well as other menopausal symptoms. Vitamins B6 and E have also been suggested, but no carefully controlled trials have been carried out. They are all available from the chemist, but the dose recommended on the packet should not be exceeded without the advice of your doctor.

Drugs your doctor may prescribe for hot flushes

- *Clonidine (Dixarit™)* Clonidine can relieve menopausal hot flushes and night sweats and is useful for women with hypertension, as it is also a treatment for high blood pressure. It is occasionally also prescribed for the prevention of migraine aggravated by the menopause. Like all drugs, it may cause side-effects, usually just feeling a little faint or tired. Less common side-effects include a dry mouth, disturbed sleep, irritability, fluid retention and nausea.

A course of clonidine should never be stopped suddenly, as it may cause a rebound rise in blood pressure. This can be prevented by reducing the dose gradually over several days or weeks.

- *Beta blockers* Doctors usually prescribe beta blockers – most commonly *atenolol (Tenormin™)* or *propranolol (Inderal™)* – for the treatment of high blood pressure or anxiety. These drugs can help reduce menopausal symptoms of hot flushes and palpitations. Common side-effects in higher doses are tiredness, cold hands and feet, disturbed sleep, and sometimes vivid dreams.

- *Progestogen* When medical reasons prevent the use of oestrogens, *norethisterone* 5 mg or *megestrol acetate* 40 mg daily are sometimes effective in relieving hot flushes.

- *The combined oral contraceptive pill* The combined oral contraceptive pill can effectively relieve hot flushes and night sweats, in addition to its contraceptive action. It is now accepted that oral contraceptives containing low doses of oestrogen are safe for healthy non-smoking women over the age of 35, right up until the time of the menopause. Their use has non-contraceptive advantages – reducing the incidence of the pre-menstrual syndrome, certain genital tract tumours, pelvic infections and anaemia. Taking the combined pill before the menopause may also increase the overall bone mass and so protect against the later development of osteoporosis.

  The combined oral contraceptive pill might be a suitable choice for some perimenopausal women who need contraception – HRT itself does not adequately prevent pregnancy (see the question on contraception in Chapter 12).

- *Selective Serotonin Reuptake Inhibitors* There is increasing evidence that drugs originally developed for the treatment of depression effectively control hot flushes. These include *venlafaxine* and *paroxetine*.

Anxiety, depression and sleepless nights
Self-help
Trying to resolve the underlying cause of the anxiety or depression is the obvious answer, but the cause is not always apparent. Exercise and diet are important for physical and mental health – the exercise

'high' can be an important morale booster. More serious problems might be resolved with the help of your partner, although it is sometimes necessary to seek professional advice if you find it difficult to cope.

Poor sleep is aggravated by alcohol and caffeine, so avoid a bedtime toddy or cup of coffee. A hot milky drink helps sleep, or you could try a hot herbal tea. Sleep-inducing herbs are elderflower, bergamot, hops, chamomile and the lime (linden) flower. These become more effective if taken over a period of time.

Drugs your doctor may prescribe
- *Sedatives and tranquillizers* Occasionally your doctor might recommend a short course of a mild sedative or tranquillizer, especially if you have difficulty sleeping or experience panic attacks. It is important that you take them exactly as prescribed, and for no longer than the recommended course: they are safe and effective for short-term use, but it is easy to become used to their effects, and even addicted to them, if they are taken for long periods.
- *Antidepressives* Depression is a common problem at the time of the menopause but HRT is only effective if the depression is the result of hormonal fluctuations. For example, hormonal changes cause night sweats, and the resulting lack of sleep can lead to depression. Treating the night sweats with HRT also treats the depression. However, hormonal changes are not the only cause, and HRT is not the only treatment. Marital difficulties, or the death of a close relative, are better treated with counselling and, if necessary, a course of antidepressives. Depression can be an illness linked to low levels of certain chemicals in the brain that are responsible for mood. Antidepressives are then necessary to restore the chemicals to their normal level. Depression is not something to be ashamed of – after all, no one is ashamed of taking iron supplements if they are anaemic. Venlafaxine and Paroxetine may treat both depression and hot flushes.

Stress incontinence

Self-help
Coughing or sneezing raises the pressure in the body, sometimes causing a small amount of urine to leak from the bladder. The main reason for this happening is that the muscles controlling the bladder

have weakened. Even before the menopause, pregnancy and childbirth stretch these muscles, and they lose their normal tone. The falling levels of oestrogen after the menopause cause the muscles to weaken further.

Exercise can improve the tone and strength of any muscle, including the muscles of the bladder. One useful exercise, each time you go to the toilet, is to try to stop the stream of urine. Squeeze the muscles to stop the flow and then relax. Repeat several times. You may find it difficult at first, but eventually it will get easier.

A similar exercise is to imagine that you are pulling the bladder up towards your head as you tighten the muscles. You can try this exercise anywhere, holding the muscles tight to a count of 10 before relaxing them. Try this exercise several times a day, whenever you remember.

Vaginal dryness and painful intercourse

Self-help

The use of water-soluble lubricants such as KY Jelly during sexual intercourse can help relieve some of the dryness. Early studies with a new compound, polycarbophil, are promising. This agent, besides acting as a lubricant, may also help prevent infections by creating a more acid environment – infections are more common after the menopause as the vaginal area becomes less acid, affecting the normal protective bacteria.

Osteoporosis

It is easier to prevent osteoporosis than to treat it, and prevention starts young. Nutritional factors and physical activity both play roles in the causes, prevention and treatment of osteoporosis.

Pregnant and nursing women are at risk of bone loss, particularly if they have repeated pregnancies, as all the calcium in the new-born infant comes from the mother. Pregnant women should make sure they have adequate amounts of calcium in their diet, taking supplements if necessary.

The risk factors for osteoporosis were discussed in Chapter 5. Clearly there is not much you can do about fixed risk factors such as your race, sex or family history, but you can change your diet.

Everyone, children and young adults included, should take more exercise. Bone is a very active substance, with a constant turnover. In osteoporosis, not enough new bone is formed to replace the amount normally broken down.

Preventing osteoporosis

Self-help
To minimize your risk of osteoporosis:

- Increase the amount of calcium in your diet, with supplements if necessary. A number of studies suggest that a good balanced diet, rich in calcium, can increase peak bone mass by 5 to 10 per cent. The bone mass established from the combination of exercise and diet could delay the average age of osteoporotic fractures by ten years.
- Eat enough to maintain a suitable body weight – thin people with a Body Mass Index (see Chapter 5) of less than 20 are at risk of osteoporosis. The ideal Body Mass Index is between 20 and 25.
- Stop smoking, or at least cut down. Long-term smoking reduces the production of oestrogen, and brings forward the age at menopause by between two and five years. Both these factors encourage the onset of osteoporosis.
- Do not drink too much alcohol – women should keep below the limit of 14 units a week (one unit = 1 glass of wine, 1 single pub measure of spirits, or 1/2 pint of beer).
- Take more exercise – diet alone is not enough. Exercise improves agility and mobility, reducing the likelihood of falls that might lead to fractures. Studies show that weight-bearing exercise positively affects bone turnover: Zulu women in South Africa have very little osteoporosis – they carry weights on their heads and walk a lot, from a very early age. This applies stress to the spine that might protect against osteoporosis. However, *excessive* exercise can cause loss of bone, so moderation is the key. A combination of exercise and calcium supplements is even more effective than either alone.
- If you are taking drugs that are known to increase bone loss, e.g. steroids or high doses of thyroxine, discuss this with your doctor.

Diet and osteoporosis: calcium
About 99 per cent of calcium is in the skeleton; the amount of calcium in the diet plays a major part in keeping the skeleton strong and healthy. The amount of bone in your body peaks around the age

of 30 and then falls gradually until the menopause. After this, the rate of fall increases as the protective effect of oestrogen is lost.

Calcium in the diet is absorbed from the gut, a process requiring vitamin D. As a woman gets older, so her daily requirement of calcium increases. The average diet provides only about 500 mg calcium each day but women after the menopause need an average of 1,500 mg to maintain the levels of calcium.

Oestrogen helps the body absorb calcium from the diet and women taking oestrogen replacement therapy require about 1,000 mg daily to keep the balance. But the absorption of calcium can be affected by the other food you eat: too much fibre can prevent calcium being taken up by the body, but lactose – the sugar in milk – enhances absorption.

Dairy foods, particularly milk, yoghurt and hard cheeses, are the major source of calcium in the diet. Consumption of these products has decreased by about 25 per cent over the last thirty years, probably because of scares about the fat content of dairy foods and heart disease. However, skimmed milk contains marginally more calcium than full fat milk, and it does not have the undesirable fat or calories. Fibre-rich foods such as spinach also contain calcium, but the body cannot absorb it so easily from non-dairy sources.

Food supplements for osteoporosis

- *Calcium supplements* The body absorbs calcium from food better than from tablets, but you can buy calcium supplements from the chemist if you are at risk of osteoporosis or do not eat much dairy produce. High doses of calcium supplements can cause constipation and flatulence, and increase the risk of developing kidney stones. If you have kidney stones or are confined to bed for any reason, you should consult your doctor before starting or continuing calcium supplements. Do not exceed 2 grams of calcium daily.

  Regular supplements of calcium become more important in later life as the body is less able to absorb calcium from the diet. Calcium can make certain drugs less effective, such as the antibiotic tetracycline. The calcium prevents the absorption of tetracycline from the stomach, so tetracycline and calcium should be taken at least three hours apart. If you are taking any other medicines, ask your doctor if there is likely to be any problem.

See Appendix 4, p. 139, for calcium supplements available in the UK.

- *Vitamin D* Aptly termed the 'sunshine vitamin', sunlight falling on the skin stimulates the production of vitamin D in the body. This vitamin helps us absorb calcium and phosphate from the food that we eat, helping the skeleton stay strong. Old people do not go outside as much as when they were younger, and this may be the reason why they absorb less calcium from their food. Getting out in the sun is the obvious solution, but housebound women eating a poor diet may benefit from supplements of vitamin D. A couple of eggs, or one ounce of margarine or butter, sardines or salmon, contain the recommended daily amount of the vitamin. A few studies have suggested that certain forms of vitamin D, in particular vitamin D3 (*calcitriol (Rocaltrol™)* can help prevent and treat osteoporosis. A combined supplement of calcium and vitamin D3 is also available (*Calcichew D3*).

Too much vitamin D can be harmful to bones: do not exceed 500 international units daily, from all sources.

Drugs

Some drugs can prevent bone loss by trying to stop the natural turnover of bone.

- *Bisphosphonates* Bisphosphonates, such as *etidronate*, are 'bone-seeking' compounds. Their more common use is for treatment of Paget's disease as they prevent the loss of bone mass. Controlled trials show that bisphosphonates may offer long-term prevention of bone loss and further fractures in those who already suffer from osteoporosis, particularly those with spinal fractures.

Etidronate is taken as a 13-week cycle: two weeks of etidronate, 400 mg daily, then 11 weeks of daily calcium supplements. The effect of etidronate lasts for several months. It is not easily absorbed into the body, and is particularly affected by iron, calcium, magnesium and aluminium, so it should be taken with water, on an empty stomach, two hours before or after eating. Side-effects include nausea, indigestion and diarrhoea, but these are rarely severe.

Alendronate is a newer bisphosphonate that also increases bone density in the spine and hip by around 8 per cent after three years' use. Despite this, the risk of fracture remains the same. Because it can cause inflammation of the oesophagus (the passage from the mouth to the stomach), the manufacturer advises that alendronate is taken with a full glass of water while standing up. It is now available as a once-weekly dose, making it easier to take. Alendronate costs about twice as much as etidronate.

Risendronate, like alendronate, is more potent than etidronate and is effective at preventing fractures in both the spine and the hip.

- *SERMS: Selective Estrogen Receptor Modulators* These compounds have been developed not only to have the actions of oestrogen on some parts of the body, such as bone, but also to avoid the unwanted effects of oestrogen on breast and the womb. Tamoxifen, used for breast cancer, was the first of these compounds to be developed but this has been refined further to Raloxifene. Raloxifene can reduce the risk of fracture of the spine by up to 50 per cent in women with established osteoporosis. However, it does not seem to have the same benefit on the prevention of other fractures, neither does it help hot flushes.
- *Calcitonin* Calcitonin is a hormone naturally produced in the body which prevents bone loss; *salcalcitonin* is a synthetic form. Some doctors recommend calcitonin as an alternative treatment for women who are unable to take oestrogen therapy. It is also used for the treatment of established osteoporosis: studies show that it can halt further loss of bone in patients who already have osteoporosis, but there is little information on whether or not this actually prevents fractures.

  It is available as a nasal spray. There are many side-effects – flushes, nausea and vomiting. The drug appears to lose effect after 12 to 16 months of use.
- *Fluoride* For some time, fluoride was thought to be a useful treatment, particularly for severe osteoporosis of the spine, but its use is now somewhat controversial. Although it does increase bone mass, some doctors think that the new bone formed is of poor quality, with little effect on preventing fractures of the spine. Furthermore, it may increase the risk of fractures of the hip and wrist. Up to one third of patients do not improve with fluoride treatment. In addition, stomach upsets and bone and joint pains are common side-effects.

  However, a recent five-year study showed that sodium fluoride can help osteoporosis if additional supplements of calcium and vitamins are taken. This regime is taken in cycles, as the drug loses its effect when taken for long periods. At present, sodium fluoride is not recommended for the treatment of osteoporosis in the UK.

- *Progestogens* Several studies suggest that progestogens alone prevent bone loss, and norethisterone in doses of 2.5–5 mg, up to 10 mg, daily may be as effective as oestrogen. This treatment is well tolerated, even in the elderly, and unlike combined HRT does not cause regular vaginal bleeding. Its widespread use cannot be advocated yet as there is little information on long-term safety.

- *Progesterone* There is some evidence from uncontrolled clinical trials that progesterone cream applied to the skin may be effective at increasing bone density and relieving menopause symptoms. However, controlled clinical trials have failed to confirm a beneficial effect. The progesterone is derived from plant sources such as the Mexican wild yam, and is identical to human progesterone. It may be suitable for women who cannot, or do not wish to, take oestrogens.

- *Phytooestrogens* These are plant substances, found in many foods, that have a similar action to oestrogen. These include soya products, chick peas, flax, whole cereals, vegetables, legumes and fruit. In the USA, the Food and Drug Administration (FDA) have approved soy protein to reduce the risk of heart disease. However, there is insufficient evidence to confirm the use of phytooestrogens in the prevention and treatment of osteoporosis, although there are anecdotal reports of efficacy.

- *Herbalism* There is some evidence that black cohosh can help menopausal symptoms. St John's wort and ginseng are also effective on depression and well-being. There are concerns that St John's wort could potentially interact with HRT, reducing its efficacy.

Self-help if you already have osteoporosis

Preventing fractures is important if you already have osteoporosis. Exercise may prevent bone loss and possibly even increase bone mass, so women should remain active and take regular exercise.

Be careful of environmental hazards that may cause falls:

- Make sure carpets fit properly, with no loose edges to trip you up.
- Wear comfortable, well-fitting shoes. Any calluses, bunions or ingrown toenails should be treated by a chiropodist.

- Do not leave any wires trailing.
- Mind the cat or dog.
- Make sure that floor surfaces are not uneven or slippery – especially when away from home.
- Clean up any spills on the floor immediately.
- Make sure that the lighting is adequate, especially on steps and stairs.
- Get a relative or friend to fit grab rails on stairs and in the bathroom, and anywhere else they might be useful.
- Do not drink too much alcohol.
- Have your vision and hearing checked regularly, especially if you notice any changes. If you need glasses, wear them, and keep them clean.
- Be very careful of uneven surfaces, etc., when you are visiting friends or other circumstances when you are away from your usual environment.
- Take extra care if you have a condition that affects your balance or posture – for example, dizziness, arthritis, stroke or Parkinson's disease.
- See your doctor if you are taking any tablets such as sedatives or tranquillizers, and some antidepressives, which could increase your likelihood of falls.

The National Osteoporosis Society

This organization was launched in 1986. It provides a forum for all aspects of osteoporosis, and regular meetings are held. It aims to bring together health professionals from the many branches of medicine involved in the management of osteoporosis: orthopaedic surgeons, endocrinologists, gynaecologists, physiotherapists and GPs. The Society provides funds for research, and a regular newsletter is sent to members, full of advice and practical ideas.

The address of the Society is: Camerton, Bath BA2 0PJ (tel: 01761 471771).

Heart disease and strokes

Conventional risk factors for heart disease and strokes include smoking, high blood pressure and high levels of cholesterol. Drugs used in the treatment and prevention of heart disease are outside the scope of this book.

Preventing heart disease

Self-help

Much of the advice to prevent osteoporosis also applies to heart disease. If you smoke, you should stop now. If you have high blood pressure or high cholesterol, you should aim to lose weight and take moderate exercise, under the supervision of your doctor.

Diet and heart disease

Obesity

Obesity, and its consequent health problems, is common in developed countries. Excess food intake is thought to be responsible for a number of diseases including heart disease, strokes, high cholesterol, high blood pressure and diabetes, to name a few.

Eating less is the only way to effectively treat obesity. The aim is to lose about 1 kg a week, which usually means limiting food intake to between 1,000 and 1,500 calories a day. Some diets promise rapid weight loss by severely restricting calorie intake. These should be avoided as they are dangerous if used for too long, and most of the weight lost is water, not fat. Dieting is not easy, but constant supervision, by either a doctor, close relatives or a slimming club, can help. Your doctor or a slimming club can also give you a diet sheet to follow. Simple changes to your diet may be enough to lose weight: switch to low-fat substitutes, avoid sugar, and eat more fibre – wholemeal bread, fresh fruit and vegetables. Alcohol is best avoided as it is high in calories. With a varied diet, vitamin and mineral supplements are unnecessary.

Drugs can be used in addition, but are not a substitute for strict dieting – some are addictive and side-effects are frequent. Operations to bypass parts of the digestive system have fallen out of favour, but in cases of extreme obesity doctors will occasionally recommend wiring the jaws together to prevent eating, or operating to make the stomach smaller. Another method is to inflate a small balloon inside the stomach. All of these can be dangerous, and although some women do lose weight, they frequently regain it when the operation is reversed.

Eating for a healthy heart

Not everyone at risk of heart disease is overweight. Even so, a change in diet, particularly if you have high cholesterol, can make a difference. Reducing the total fat intake is important, especially saturated fats from meat and dairy products. Use skimmed milk and low-fat substitutes for butter and cheese. Eat more chicken and fish, limiting red meats to once or twice a week. Why not try a few vegetarian alternatives? Try to avoid foods with a high sugar content, such as biscuits, cakes and puddings, as they are usually also high in fat.

Exercise for a healthy heart and strong bones

It is never too late to start exercise. Even if you already have osteoporosis or heart disease, you can strengthen the bone and heart muscle that remains. There is increasing evidence that physical activity and physical fitness reduces heart disease, stroke, hypertension, obesity, diabetes, cancer of the colon, and depression. Exercise has a stimulant effect on well-being, sleep and physical energy. The body's own natural painkillers and antidepressives are released, resulting in the 'runner's high' – a feeling of well-being and euphoria following exercise. Maintaining physical activity and taking regular exercise reduces the rate of bone loss, protecting against heart disease. There are some who even believe that exercise may prevent premature ageing of the brain.

The simplest way of taking regular exercise is to include it as part of your daily routine – walking is the easiest exercise to do, but try to walk at a brisk pace for maximum effect. Walk instead of taking the car to the local shops; climb the stairs rather than using the lift. If you travel further afield, consider investing in a bicycle. Cycling does not put any strain on the joints, and if you suffer from arthritis, cycling will help make it easier to walk.

Any exercise programme should be developed to allow a gradual build-up of muscle strength and endurance. Exercise at least three or four times a week, for at least 30 minutes, to achieve maximum benefit.

Any aerobic exercise, such as walking, jogging, swimming or riding a bicycle, sufficient to increase the average resting heart rate by about 70 per cent, will help protect against heart disease.

To estimate this, you must first work out your maximum heart rate by subtracting your age from 220. For example, if you are 50, your predicted maximum heart rate is 170 beats per minute. To work out the necessary rate when exercising, multiply the predicated maximum rate by 0.7. The sum (assuming your age is 50) will look like this:

$$(220 - 50) \times 0.7 = 119$$

Using the above example, the heart rate to aim for when exercising will be 119 beats per minute.

To check your heart rate, feel the radial pulse on the thumb side of the inner wrist, using the first two fingers of the other hand. Count the number of beats over a 10-second interval and multiply by 6 to calculate the number of beats per minute.

Exercises to protect against bone loss need to be weight-bearing, so swimming is not very effective but walking, jogging and weight training are.

The best routine is to do some simple stretching exercises for 10 to 15 minutes every day, combined with aerobic exercises for 30 minutes every other day.

Exercise is not a panacea. However, combined with an appropriate lifestyle and balanced diet, it can substantially improve energy levels and general health. Having read about the effects of HRT on heart disease and osteoporosis, there is the temptation to believe that HRT is a substitute for exercise and diet. Do not be misled; the reverse is the true story – exercise and a healthy diet give additional benefits and might, for some women, be an effective alternative to hormone therapy.

Summary

- There are many alternatives to HRT for the treatment of menopausal symptoms.
- Diet and exercise play an important role in preventing osteoporosis and heart disease – it is never too late to make changes.

11

The Future

An enormous amount of research had been published in recent years. This has led to greater awareness of the short- and long-term consequences of the menopause, and the role of HRT. However, it has taken a long time for the information from specialists to reach the family doctor; sometimes the results of studies are published in the popular press before they have reached the medical literature, and the 'facts' are not always accurate. This has resulted in confusion about the true effects of HRT, which only time and accurate information will resolve.

Many questions remain unanswered, and long-term clinical trials are vital to help us understand the risks and benefits of HRT. Interpreting the results of studies can be confusing. Many women now approaching the menopause took oral contraceptives containing high doses of oestrogen, unlike the low dose pills currently used. This may in itself have long-term effects on heart disease, the results only becoming apparent many years later. Only studies properly designed to screen out these confounding problems will reveal the answers.

The role of research

Women who choose to take hormones tend to be more health conscious and have a higher standard of living, which may contribute to their lower coronary risk.

This has meant that the true benefits of HRT may have been overestimated – a view supported by the results of recent studies.

The Women's Health Initiative (WHI) study included over 16,000 post-menopausal women who were taking either conjugated equine oestrogens 0.625 mg plus medroxyprogesterone (MPA) 2.5 mg (similar to Premique in the UK) daily or placebo (dummy treatment). Although the study was planned to run for over eight years, it was stopped after five years because the number of cases of breast cancer in the HRT users had reached a prespecified safety limit. The results suggested that for 10,000 women taking HRT each year compared to non-users there would be an extra eight cases of

118

breast cancer, seven heart attacks, eight strokes and eight lung clots. On the positive side, there would be six fewer bowel cancers and five fewer hip fractures. Although the increased risk of breast cancer was previously known, the effect of HRT on heart disease was surprising, as it contrasted with what is known about the action of oestrogens. What has not been considered in the interpretations of the results of this study is that it is possible that medroxyprogesterone acetate, the progestogen used, could have a negative effect, countering the benefits of oestrogen. In line with this, the oestrogen-alone arm of the study has not been discontinued and we will have to wait a few more years to know whether it is oestrogen or the particular progestogen used in the study that is responsible for these findings.

It is unfortunate that another large UK study was terminated following the reports of the WHI study. The Women's International Study of Long Duration Oestrogen after Menopause (WISDOM) study was a long-term study of the effects of HRT on heart disease, osteoporosis and breast cancer. However, the WISDOM study used the same combination of oestrogen and progestogen as was used in the WHI study, leading to safety concerns about continuing the study.

This is unfortunate, as several different factors could have been studied in the UK research. However, now more than ever, research must be undertaken on different HRT combinations, particularly using human oestrogens and different progestogens. Although the benefits of HRT on bowel cancer and osteoporosis have been confirmed in both these and other studies, the true risks of HRT remain unclear. Studies also need to confirm the suspected benefits of HRT on other conditions such as dementia and cataracts.

There appears little problem with short-term use of HRT for a few years in perimenopausal women. Until hard evidence is available, long-term HRT depends on the individual needs and potential risks of each woman. The dose of HRT should be kept to the minimum necessary to control symptoms or protect bone.

Some women continue to produce sufficient oestrogen after the menopause and would not necessarily gain any benefit from taking HRT. Accurate and cheap tests to measure bone loss and to assess the risk of heart disease could be used in large screening programmes to help identify those women who would benefit most from hormone replacement therapy.

THE FUTURE

If it is ever possible to develop the ideal hormone replacement therapy, it will:

- effectively suppress hot flushes, night sweats and other symptoms of oestrogen deficiency;
- prevent and treat osteoporosis;
- protect against heart disease and stroke;
- protect against cancer;
- have no side-effects.

We live in hope!

12

Questions and Answers

Do I need contraception if I am taking HRT?
HRT does not restore fertility so you cannot become pregnant if you start HRT several years after the menopause. However, it is important to realize that most types of HRT are not contraceptive, and if you start HRT before your periods have naturally ceased there is a risk of pregnancy. For this reason, you should continue using non-hormonal contraception until at least one year after the menopause if you were already over the age of 50, or for two years if you were under 50. About 80 per cent of women are post-menopause by the age of 54.

Alternatively, you could take the combined oral contraceptive (COC) containing the lowest dose of oestrogen. The new low dose combined pills can be prescribed for non-smoking women up to the time of the menopause. It will mask the symptoms of the menopause as it artificially creates regular 'periods' each month during the pill-free week. The pill is stopped at the age of 50 to assess if the woman has reached the menopause. It is then possible to switch to HRT if necessary.

The progestogen-only pill (POP) becomes more effective as you become less fertile – in women over the age of 40, the combined pill and the POP are equally effective. Unlike the combined pill, you can take the POP if you smoke, or if you have been advised not to take contraceptive oestrogens. Since there is no upper age limit, you can take it right up to the menopause. However, it is unlikely that the amount of progestogen is sufficient to prevent hot flushes and night sweats.

Use of the POP together with HRT has not been properly evaluated and is not generally recommended for most women.

The Mirena intrauterine system has the advantage of being a highly effective method of contraception and reduces menstrual bleeding. It is used in several countries as the progestogen component of HRT, although it is not licensed for this purpose in the UK at the time of writing.

You should discuss contraception with your doctor or local family planning clinic.

I have been taking HRT for several months, but do not feel any better.

There are three possible reasons for this which you should discuss with your doctor:

1 The symptoms are not due to the hormonal changes of the menopause.
2 The dose of oestrogen is not enough, and a higher dose may be necessary.
3 If you are taking HRT in tablet form, it is possible that not enough gets into the bloodstream to be effective. Changing to skin patches or implants might make a difference.

My doctor said I could not take the pill because I smoke. Can I take HRT?

The oestrogens used in hormone replacement therapy are completely different to those used in the oral contraceptive pill. First, HRT uses 'naturally' occurring oestrogens, rather than synthetic; second, the dose of oestrogen required is much lower than that necessary for contraception. For these reasons, unlike the oral contraceptive pill, HRT can be taken by women who smoke, although it is always better to quit the habit.

Can I take HRT if I have high blood pressure?

High blood pressure should be investigated and controlled (losing weight, stopping smoking, drug treatments) before starting treatment. Some doctors prefer to prescribe patches or implants rather than tablets; this is theoretically less likely to affect changes in the liver thought to be involved in hypertension.

If you develop high blood pressure when taking HRT, it is not always necessary to stop treatment. A few women develop high blood pressure because they are sensitive to oral oestrogens; changing to an alternative route may be sufficient.

A year ago I had a heart attack. Now I am getting menopausal symptoms and would like to start HRT.

Studies show that certain types of HRT do not protect against heart disease (those containing conjugated equine oestrogens and medroxy-progesterone acetate). It is not known if the same applies to other types of HRT. If you have previously had angina or a heart attack, you should see your doctor to discuss the possible benefits and risks of HRT for you, as well as considering non-hormonal alternatives.

Does HRT interfere with any other tablets I take?
HRT is rarely affected by any other medication you might take. A few medicines interact with the way your liver deals with the HRT, which can then lead to irregular bleeding or a return of the menopausal symptoms. This is more likely to happen if you take tablets for HRT than if you are using patches or implants. Medicines which might have this effect are some of those usually prescribed for epilepsy, such as *phenytoin* or *carbamazepine*. Rarely, certain antibiotics have a similar effect. The herbal treatment St John's wort may also interact with HRT. Always check with your doctor if you have any doubts about what you are taking.

What if I forget my HRT for a few days?
You may lose the effect of the HRT if you forget to take it, which can cause irregular bleeding or the return of symptoms. Start taking the HRT, as normal, as soon as you remember, but stick to the usual dose – do not try and catch up on the tablets you have missed.

If you are a few days late starting a course of the progestogen tablets, start them immediately and take them for the same number of days you normally take each month. Check with your doctor about when to take the progestogen course the following month. If you are more than a couple of weeks late, skip that course, and take it the following month, as usual.

A stomach upset with diarrhoea or vomiting may stop tablets of HRT being absorbed, so again, you might get some irregular bleeding or return of the symptoms. Absorption of the hormones by non-oral routes of HRT will not be affected by vomiting or diarrhoea.

I am 62 and my last period was when I was 51. I would like to take HRT but do I have to have a monthly period again?
Many of the regimens for HRT in premenopausal women result in monthly 'periods', stimulated by the cycle of progestogens. This is necessary because most pre-menopausal women still have some hormone activity of their own and imposing a 'period-free' regimen of HRT often results in erratic bleeding. This settles after the menopause and so post-menopausal women can take combined oestrogen and progestogen every day, with no monthly 'period'.

Will I put on weight?
All studies show that all women gain weight as they get older. Most women on HRT do not gain more weight compared to non-HRT users, and some even lose weight. However, particularly in the early stages of treatment, fluid retention can be a problem, although this usually settles after a few months. If not, the dose of oestrogen may be too high, and cutting down the dose can relieve the symptoms. A small number of women taking HRT experience a dramatic weight gain and have to stop treatment.

Will HRT help my sex life?
It is natural for sex to become less frequent as you grow older. Depression and illness both play their part, but menopausal symptoms can be the final straw. Night sweats, tiredness and vaginal dryness do not exactly set the scene for passion. If the problem is due to the symptoms of oestrogen withdrawal, HRT will make a difference. Some doctors recommend testosterone implants to improve libido. However, HRT cannot improve the problems of an already difficult relationship.

I am going into hospital soon, for an operation. Will I have to stop HRT?
Doctors generally advise women to stop HRT about 4–6 weeks before an operation that will result in a period of immobility. This usually means major surgery or leg surgery. This is because the combination of oestrogen and immobility make the blood more likely to clot, increasing the risk of thrombosis of the leg (DVT) or a clot on the lung. You can start HRT again as soon as you are up and about.

I have had oestrogen implants replaced every six months, but when I went for my recent six-monthly visit, I decided to stop the treatment. However, my doctor said I had to continue the monthly courses of progestogen, possibly for another 18 months. Why?
The effects of oestrogen implants last for much longer after stopping treatment than tablets or patches. This means that the lining of the uterus continues to be stimulated and could, in rare cases, turn cancerous. To prevent this happening, doctors suggest that you continue the monthly course of progestogen, until it ceases to stimulate bleeding. In some cases, this may be up to two years from the date of the last implant.

Do I have to take HRT for the rest of my life?
Most women only take HRT for a couple of years to treat hot flushes and night sweats. Women at risk of osteoporosis should consider taking HRT for the rest of their lives in order to gain full benefit.

Can I take HRT indefinitely?
Some women feel so well on HRT that they are loathe to stop treatment – particularly if they have had a hysterectomy. The major concern about long-term therapy (more than five years' continued use) is the increased risk of breast cancer. If you accept this risk, there is no reason to discontinue HRT.

How do I stop taking HRT?
Stopping HRT abruptly can result in a return of the symptoms. To prevent this, HRT should be tailed off gradually over two to three months under the supervision of your doctor.

What happens when I stop taking HRT?
If hot flushes and night sweats continue or return a couple of months after stopping HRT, you may decide to take a further course of HRT for several months before tailing off the treatment again. Symptoms such as a dry or painful vagina can be controlled with local oestrogens inserted into the vagina.

Appendix 1
Related Reading

Coping with the Menopause, Janet Horwood, Sheldon Press, 2001
ISBN: 0–85969–834–3
Price: £6.99

Living with Osteoporosis, Dr Joan Gomez, Sheldon Press, 2000
ISBN: 0–85969–838–6
Price: £6.99

Appendix 2
Useful Addresses

When writing to any of these organizations, please enclose an SAE.

The Amarant Trust
Head Office and Clinic:
The Gainsborough Clinic
80 Lambeth Road
London SE1 7PW
Tel: 020 7401 3855
Helpline: 01293 413000 (11 a.m.–6 p.m. Mon–Fri)

Family Planning Association
2–12 Pentonville Road
London N1 9FP
Tel: 020 7837 5432
Helpline: 0845 310 1334 (9 a.m.–7 p.m. Mon–Fri)
Website: www.fpa.org.uk

The National Osteoporosis Society
Camerton
Bath BA2 0PJ
Tel: 01761 471771
Helpline: 0845 450 0203
Website: www.nos.org.uk

Women's Health Concern
PO Box 2126
Marlow
Bucks SL7 2RY
Tel: 01628 488065
Helpline: 01628 483612

The City of London Migraine Clinic
22 Charterhouse Square
London EC1M 6DX
Tel: 020 7251 3322
Website: www.colmc.org.uk

Appendix 3
Sex Hormone Therapies

Systemic (for flushes, sweats, etc., and protection against osteoporosis)

Oestrogen only (for women who have had a hysterectomy, otherwise additional progestogen is necessary)

Tablets

Adgyn Estro (Strakan)
- oestradiol 2 mg (white)
1 tablet daily.

Climaval (Novartis)
- oestradiol valerate 1 mg (grey-blue); or 2 mg (blue)
1–2 mg daily.

Elleste Solo (Pharmacia)
- oestradiol 1 mg (white); or 2 mg (orange)
1–2 mg daily.

Harmogen (Pharmacia)
- estropipate 1.5 mg (peach)
1–2 tablets daily.

Hormonin (Shire)
- oestriol 0.27 mg, oestrone 1.4 mg, oestradiol 0.6 mg (pink)
1–2 tablets daily taken continuously or cyclically.

Premarin (Wyeth)
- conjugated oestrogens 0.625 mg (maroon); or 1.25 mg (yellow)
1 tablet daily.

Progynova (Schering HC)
- oestradiol valerate 1 mg (beige); or 2 mg (blue)
1 tablet daily.

Zumenon (Solvay)
- oestradiol 1 mg (white); 2 mg (red)
1–2 tablets daily.

Skin patches

Dermestril (Straken)
- oestradiol 25; or 50; or 100 microgram patches
1 patch replaced every 3–4 days.
or
Dermestril Septem
- oestradiol 50; or 100 microgram patches
1 patch replaced every 7 days.

Elleste Solo MX40 (Pharmacia)
- oestradiol 40 microgram patch
1 patch replaced every 3–4 days.
or
Elleste Solo MX80
- oestradiol 80 microgram patch
1 patch replaced every 3–4 days.

Estraderm MX (Novartis)
- oestradiol 25; or 50; or 75; or 100 microgram patches
1 patch replaced every 3–4 days.
or
Estraderm TTS
- oestradiol 25; or 50; or 100 microgram patches
1 patch replaced every 3–4 days.

Evorel (Janssen-Cilag)
- oestradiol 25; or 50; or 75; or 100 microgram patches
1 patch replaced every 3–4 days.

Fematrix (Solvay)
- oestradiol 40; or 80 microgram patches
1 patch replaced every 3–4 days.

Femseven (Merck)
- oestradiol 50; or 75; or 100 microgram patches
1 patch replaced every 7 days.

Menorest (Novartis)
- oestradiol 37.5; or 50; or 75 microgram patches
1 patch replaced every 3–4 days.

Progynova TS (Schering HC)
- oestradiol 50; or 100 microgram patches
1 patch replaced every 7 days.

Gel

Oestrogel (Hoescht)
- oestradiol 1.5 mg
2 measures once daily applied to arms, shoulders or inner thighs; increase to 4 measures daily if inadequate response after 1 month.

Sandrena (Organon)
- oestradiol 0.5 mg, 1 mg in single dose units
Initially 1 mg applied once daily to the right or left thigh, on alternate days. Adjust after 2–3 cycles within range 0.5–1.5 mg daily.

Nasal spray

Aerodiol (Servier)
- oestradiol hemihydrate 150 microgram per spray
1–4 sprays daily.

Systemic vaginal ring

Menoring (Galen)
- oestradiol 50 microgram per 24 hours
1 ring inserted into upper third of the vagina. This should be replaced with a new ring after 3 months.

Progestogen

Tablets
Adgyn Medro (Strakan)
- medroxyprogesterone acetate 5 mg (white)

Duphaston–HRT (Solvay)
- dydrogesterone 10 mg (yellow)

Micronor–HRT (Janssen-Cilag)
- norethisterone 1 mg (white)

Provera (Pharmacia)
- medroxyprogesterone acetate 2.5 mg (orange); 5 mg (blue); or 10 mg (white)

Suppositories/pessaries
Cyclogest (Shire)
- progesterone 200 mg; 400 mg by vagina or rectum

Vaginal gel
Crinone (Serono)
- progesterone 4%

Oestrogen/progestogen combinations

Tablets
Adgyn Combi (Straken)
- oestradiol 2 mg (white)
- oestradiol 2 mg + norethisterone 1 mg (pink)
1 daily without a break starting with white.

Climagest (Novartis)
- oestradiol valerate 1 mg (grey-blue)
- oestradiol valerate 1 mg + norethisterone 1 mg (white)
or
- oestradiol valerate 2 mg (blue)
- oestradiol valerate 2 mg + norethisterone 1 mg (yellow)
1 daily without a break starting with grey-blue or blue.

Cyclo-Progynova (Viatris)
• oestradiol valerate 1 mg (beige)
• oestradiol valerate 1 mg + levonorgestrel 0.25 mg (brown)
or
• oestradiol valerate 2 mg (white)
• oestradiol valerate 2 mg + levonorgestrel 0.5 mg (brown)
1 oestradiol tablet daily for 11 days then 1 combined tablet daily for
10 days followed by 7 tablet-free days.

Elleste Duet (Pharmacia)
• oestradiol 1 mg (white)
• oestradiol 1 mg + norethisterone acetate 1 mg (green)
or
• oestradiol 2 mg (orange)
• oestradiol 2 mg + norethisterone acetate 1 mg (grey)
1 daily starting with white or orange tablets.

Femoston 1/10 (Solvay)
• oestradiol 1 mg (white)
• oestradiol 1 mg + dydrogesterone 10 mg (grey)
or
Femoston 2/10
• oestradiol 2 mg (red)
• oestradiol 2 mg + dydrogesterone 10 mg (yellow)
or
Femoston 2/20
• oestradiol 2 mg (red)
• oestradiol 2 mg + dydrogesterone 20 mg (blue)
1 tablet daily without a break starting with white or red.

Nuvelle (Schering HC)
• oestradiol valerate 2 mg (white)
• oestradiol valerate 2 mg + levonorgestrel 75 micrograms (pink)
1 white tablet daily for 16 days, then 1 pink tablet daily for 12 days.

Premique Cycle (Wyeth)
• conjugated oestrogens 0.625 mg (white)
• conjugated oestrogens 0.625 mg + medroxyprogesterone acetate
  10 mg (green)
1 white tablet daily for 14 days, then 1 green tablet daily for next 14
days.

Prempak-C (Wyeth)
- conjugated oestrogens 0.625 mg (maroon); or 1.25 mg (yellow)
- norgestrel 0.15 mg (brown)

1 maroon (or yellow) tab for 16 days then 1 maroon (or yellow) tab + 1 brown tab for 12 days.

Trisequens (Novo Nordisk)
- oestradiol 2 mg (12 blue)
- oestradiol 2 mg + norethisterone acetate 1 mg (10 white)
- oestradiol 1 mg (6 red)

or

Trisequens Forte
- oestradiol 4 mg (12 yellow)
- oestradiol 4 mg + norethisterone acetate 1 mg (10 white)
- oestradiol 1 mg (6 red)

1 daily without break in medication starting with blue or yellow and following sequence.

Patches/tablets

Estrapak (Novartis)
- oestradiol 50 microgram patch
- norethisterone acetate 1 mg (red tablet)

Replace patch every 3–4 days using a different site (2 patches every week); 1 tablet daily on days 15–26 of each 28 days of oestrogen replacement.

Evorel-Pak (Janssen-Cilag)
- oestradiol 50 microgram patch
- norethisterone 1 mg (white tablet)

1 patch replaced every 3–4 days; 1 tablet daily on days 15–26 of each cycle.

Femapak 40 (Solvay)
- oestradiol 40 microgram patch
- dydrogesterone 10 mg (white tablet)

or

Femapak 80
- oestradiol 80 microgram patch
- dydrogesterone 10 mg (white tablet)

1 patch replaced every 3–4 days; 1 tablet daily for last 14 days of each cycle.

Cyclical combined patches

Estracombi (Novartis)
- oestradiol 50 microgram patch
- oestradiol 50 microgram + norethisterone 250 microgram combined patch

Apply oestradiol patch twice weekly for two weeks, followed by combined patch twice weekly for two weeks.

Evorel Sequi (Janssen-Cilag)
- oestradiol 50 microgram patch
- oestradiol 50 micrograms + norethisterone 170 microgram combined patch

1 oestradiol patch every 3–4 days for the first two weeks (2 patches every week), 1 combined patch every 3–4 days for the next two weeks.

Femseven Sequi (Merck)
- oestradiol 50 microgram patch
- oestradiol 50 microgram + levonorgestrel 10 microgram combined patch

1 oestradiol patch every 7 days for the first two weeks, 1 combined patch every 7 days for the next two weeks.

Sequential oestrogen/progestogen combinations: quarterly bleed

Tablets

Tridestra (Sanofi Winthrop)
- oestradiol valerate 2 mg (70 white)
- oestradiol valerate 2 mg + medroxyprogesterone acetate 20 mg (14 blue)
- placebo (7 yellow)

1 white tablet daily for 70 days, then 1 blue tablet daily for 14 days, then 1 yellow tablet for 7 days.

Continuous oestrogen/progestogen combinations: 'period'-free

Tablets

Climesse (Novartis)
- oestradiol valerate 2 mg; norethisterone 0.7 mg (pink)
1 tablet daily.

Elleste Duet Conti (Pharmacia)
- oestradiol 2 mg; norethisterone 1 mg (grey)
1 tablet daily.

Femoston Conti (Solvay)
- oestradiol 1 mg; dydrogesterone 5 mg (pink)
1 tablet daily.

Indivina (Orion)
- oestradiol 1 mg; medroxyprogesterone acetate 2.5 mg (white)
or
- oestradiol 1 mg; medroxyprogesterone acetate 5 mg (white)
or
- oestradiol 2 mg; medroxyprogesterone acetate 5 mg (white)
1 tablet daily.

Kliofem (Novo Nordisk)
- oestradiol 2 mg; norethisterone acetate 1 mg (yellow)
1 tablet daily.

Kliovance (Novo Nordisk)
- oestradiol 1 mg; norethisterone acetate 0.5 mg (white)
1 tablet daily.

Nuvelle Continuous (Schering HC)
- oestradiol hemihydrate 2 mg; norethisterone acetate 1 mg (pink)
1 tablet daily.

Premique (Wyeth)
- conjugated oestrogens 0.625 mg; medroxyprogesterone acetate 5 mg (blue)
1 tablet daily.

Continuous combined patches

Evorel Conti (Janssen-Cilag)
- oestradiol 50 micrograms + norethisterone 170 microgram combined patch

1 oestradiol patch every 3–4 days (2 patches every week).

Femseven Conti (Merck)
- oestradiol 50 micrograms + levonorgestrel 7 microgram combined patch

1 oestradiol patch every 7 days (1 patch every week).

Tibolone

Livial (Organon)
- tibolone 2.5 mg (white)

1 tablet daily.

Local oestrogens for vaginal symptoms

Creams and pessaries

Ortho-Gynest (Janssen-Cilag)
- oestriol 0.5 mg (pessary); or oestriol 0.01% (cream)

1 pessary or applicatorful every evening; maintenance, 1 pessary or applicatorful twice weekly.

Ovestin (Organon)
- oestriol 1 mg (white)

0.5–3 mg daily for up to 1 month then 0.5–1 mg daily.
or
- oestriol 0.1% (cream)

1 applicator dose intravaginally daily for 3 weeks; maintenance, 1 applicator dose twice a week.

Premarin vaginal cream (Wyeth)
- conjugated oestrogens 0.625 mg per gram (cream)

1–2 g daily topically/intravaginally using calibrated applicator for 3 weeks followed by 1 week's rest.

Tampovagan (Co-Pharma)
- stilboestrol 0.5 mg + lactic acid 5% (pessary)

2 high into the vagina at night for 2–3 weeks.

Vagifem (Novo Nordisk)
- oestradiol 25 micrograms (vaginal tablet)

1 intravaginally daily for 2 weeks, then 1 twice per week.

Ring

Estring (Pharmacia)
- oestradiol hemihydrate 7.5 micrograms/24 hours (vaginal ring)

1 ring inserted high into vagina and worn continuously for 3 months.
Replace with new ring at 3-month intervals.

Appendix 4
Other Medicaments Indicated for Osteoporosis

Anabolic steroids

Deca-Durabolin (Organon)
- nandrolone decanoate

50 mg intramuscular injection every three weeks.

Calcitonin

Calsynar (RPR)
- salcalcitonin 100 i.u./ml; 200 i.u./ml

100 i.u. daily by subcutaneous or intramuscular injection. Patients should also receive 600 mg elemental calcium and 400 units vitamin D daily.

Miacalcic (Novartis)
- salcalcitonin 100 i.u./ml

100 i.u. daily by subcutaneous or intramuscular injection. Patients should also receive 600 mg elemental calcium and 400 units vitamin D daily.
also
- salcalcitonin 200 i.u. per spray metered dose nasal spray

1 spray daily. Maintain adequate calcium and vitamin D intake.

Calcium supplements

Cacit (Procter & Gamble)
- calcium carbonate 1.25 mg (= 12.5 mmol calcium) (pink effervescent tablet)

1–3 tablets daily in water.

Calcichew (Shire)
- calcium carbonate 1.25 g (= 500 mg calcium) (white chewable tablet)

or
Calcichew Forte
- calcium carbonate 2.5 g (= 1 g calcium) (white chewable tablet)

2.5–3.75 g daily.

Calcidrink (Shire)
- calcium carbonate 2.52 g (= 1000 mg calcium) (granules)

1 daily in water.

Calcium-Sandoz (Alliance)
- calcium glubionate 1.09 g; calcium lactobionate 0.727 g per 5 ml providing 108 mg calcium (2.7 mmol) (syrup)

55–75 ml daily.

Ossopan 800 (Sanofi-Synthelabo)
- hydroxyapatite compound 830 mg tablet (buff tablet)

4–8 tablets daily in divided doses before meals

or

Ossopan granules
- hydroxyapatite compound 3.32 g

cocoa-flavoured granules in sachet

1–2 sachets daily with or before food.

Ostram (Merck)
- calcium phosphate 3.3 g (= 1.2 g calcium) (powder)

1 sachet daily in water.

Sandocal 400 (Novartis Consumer)
- calcium lactate gluconate 930 mg, calcium carbonate 700 mg (= 400 mg calcium), citric acid 1.189 g (white effervescent tablet)

or

Sandocal 1000
- calcium lactate gluconate 2.327 g, calcium carbonate 1.75 g (= 1000 mg calcium), citric acid 2.973 g (white effervescent tablet)

1–2 g daily in water

or

Calcium Sandoz syrup
- calcium glubionate 3.27 g, calcium lactobionate 2.17 g per 15 ml

55–75 ml daily.

Calcium/vitamin D supplements

Adcal-D3 (Strakan)
- calcium carbonate 1.5 g (= 600 mg calcium); vitamin D3 400 i.u. (chewable tablet)

1 twice daily.

Cacit D3 (Procter & Gamble)
- calcium carbonate 1.25 g (= 500 mg calcium); vitamin D3 440 i.u. (effervescent granules)

1–2 sachets daily.

Calceos (Provalis)
- calcium carbonate 1.25 g (= 500 mg calcium); vitamin D3 400 i.u. (chewable tablet)

1 twice daily.

Calcichew D3 (Shire)
- calcium carbonate 1.25 g (= 500 mg calcium); vitamin D3 200 i.u. (chewable tablet)

or

Calcichew D3 Forte
- calcium carbonate 1.25 g (= 500 mg calcium); vitamin D3 400 i.u. (white chewable tablet)

2 tablets daily.

Vitamin D analogue

Rocaltrol (Roche)
- calcitriol 0.25 micrograms (red/white capsule)

1 capsule twice daily.

Bisphosphonate/calcium

Didronel PMO (Procter & Gamble)
- etridonate disodium 400 mg (14 white tablets)
- calcium carbonate 1250 mg (4 x 19 pink effervescent tablets)

1 white tablet daily taken with water followed by 1 pink tablet daily in water for 76 days.

Bisphosphonate

Actonel (Procter & Gamble)
- risendronate sodium 5 mg (yellow)

1 tablet daily.

Fosomax (M.S.D.)
- alendronate sodium (= 5 mg alendronic acid) (white tablets)

1–2 daily in the morning with a full glass of tap water, 30 mins before food, drink or other oral medication. Remain upright for 30 mins after dose.

or

Fosomax Once Weekly (M.S.D.)
- alendronate sodium (= 70 mg alendronic acid) (white tablets) 1 weekly.

Selective Oestrogen Receptor Modulator

Evista (Lilly)
- raloxifene hydrochloride 60 mg (white tablets) 1 daily.

Appendix 5
Should you take HRT?

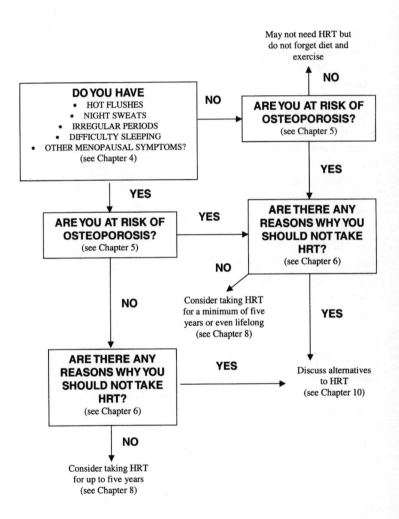

May not need HRT but
do not forget diet and
exercise

NO

DO YOU HAVE
- HOT FLUSHES
- NIGHT SWEATS
- IRREGULAR PERIODS
- DIFFICULTY SLEEPING
- OTHER MENOPAUSAL SYMPTOMS?
(see Chapter 4)

NO

ARE YOU AT RISK OF OSTEOPOROSIS?
(see Chapter 5)

YES

YES

ARE YOU AT RISK OF OSTEOPOROSIS?
(see Chapter 5)

YES

ARE THERE ANY REASONS WHY YOU SHOULD NOT TAKE HRT?
(see Chapter 6)

NO

Consider taking HRT
for a minimum of five
years or even lifelong
(see Chapter 8)

YES

NO

ARE THERE ANY REASONS WHY YOU SHOULD NOT TAKE HRT?
(see Chapter 6)

YES

Discuss alternatives
to HRT
(see Chapter 10)

NO

Consider taking HRT
for up to five years
(see Chapter 8)

Index

144